Nursing the Cardiac Patient

Nursing the Cardiac Patient

Edited by

Melanie Humphreys

Director of Postgraduate & Post-qualifying Studies
School of Nursing and Midwifery, Faculty of Health
Keele University, Keele, UK

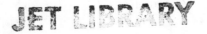
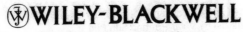
WILEY-BLACKWELL
A John Wiley & Sons, Ltd., Publication

This edition first published 2011
© 2011 by Blackwell Publishing Ltd

Blackwell Publishing was acquired by John Wiley & Sons in February 2007.
Blackwell's publishing program has been merged with Wiley's global Scientific,
Technical and Medical business to form Wiley-Blackwell.

Registered office: John Wiley & Sons, Ltd, The Atrium, Southern Gate, Chichester,
West Sussex, PO19 8SQ, UK

Editorial offices: 9600 Garsington Road, Oxford, OX4 2DQ, UK
The Atrium, Southern Gate, Chichester, West Sussex, PO19 8SQ,
UK
2121 State Avenue, Ames, Iowa 50014-8300, USA

For details of our global editorial offices, for customer services and for information
about how to apply for permission to reuse the copyright material in this book
please see our website at www.wiley.com/wiley-blackwell.

Library of Congress Cataloging-in-Publication Data
Nursing the cardiac patient / edited by Melanie Humphreys.
    p. ; cm. – (Essential clinical skills for nurses)
  Includes bibliographical references and index.
  ISBN-13: 978-1-4051-8430-4 (pbk. : alk. paper)
  ISBN-10: 1-4051-8430-2 (pbk. : alk. paper)   1. Heart-Diseases-Nursing-
Great Britian.   2. Heart-Diseases-Patients-Nursing-Great Britian.   I.
Humphreys, Melanie.   II. Series: Essential clinical skills for nurses.
  [DNLM: 1. Cardiovascular Diseases-nursing-Great Britain.   2. Nursing
Care-methods-Great Britain.   WY 152.5]
  RC674.N89 2011
  616.1'20231-dc23

                                                              2011015207

A catalogue record for this book is available from the British Library.

This book is published in the following electronic formats: ePDF 9781444346121;
ePub 9781444346138; Mobi 9781444346145

Set in 9/12.5 pt Interstate Light by Toppan Best-set Premedia Limited
Printed and bound in Malaysia by Vivar Printing Sdn Bhd

1 2011

Contents

Contributor Biographies

Editor

Melanie Humphreys
Director of Postgraduate and Post-qualifying Studies, Senior Lecturer in Nursing
MSc Research Methodology, MA Medical Ethics and Law, BSc (Hons) Educational Studies (Nursing), RNT, RGN, ONC, ENB 124, ENB 998
Melanie is currently Director of Postgraduate Studies and Post-qualifying Studies, at the School of Nursing and Midwifery at Keele University. She has many years' experience in nursing and teaching within cardiac care and emergency care. She currently undertakes a role as educational consultant to the Resuscitation Council (UK) on their generic instructor courses (GIC) delivered across the UK, and is an advanced life support (ALS) instructor.

Consultant Editor

Dr Dominic Cox
Consultant Interventional Cardiologist
MBChB, BSc (Hons) Physiol, MRCP
Dominic has worked as a consultant interventional cardiologist at Northampton General Hospital since 2004. His specialist interests are in coronary intervention, general cardiology and bradycardia pacing. He initially studied human physiology and worked on diving and survival physiology at the National Hyperbaric centre. He then trained in medicine in Aberdeen and undertook specialist training in cardiology in the north east of England. He undertakes the role of medical director and instructor on both ALS and GIC courses.

Contributors

Lisa Cooper
Advanced Nurse Practitioner - Sister, Emergency Department
MSc Advanced Clinical Nursing Practice, BN Hons, ALS(I)
Lisa has worked in A&E for 20 years, the past 10 years as a sister at Walsall Manor Hospital. She is an Advanced Nurse Practitioner and an ALS instructor. She has worked with the British Paralympic swimming team and attended both the Sydney and Athens Paralympic games as part of the team, and has

also attended many European Championships. She currently works part time in clinical informatics as a business change facilitator, while maintaining her role in A&E.

Brenda Cottam
Assistant Director of Education, BASICS Education Scotland
RGN, ENB 182, DPSN, DipIMC (RCSEd), PGCert Med Ed
Brenda is currently working as the Assistant Director of Education with BASICS Education Scotland and is a founder nurse member of the Faculty of Pre-Hospital Care. BASICS Education Scotland provides education and training for healthcare professionals involved in pre-hospital immediate medical care across Scotland, mostly GPs and nurses working in remote, rural and island practice areas. Brenda has a background in anaesthesia and cardiac critical care nursing in both the UK and USA, and held a resuscitation officer position in Tayside for eight years. Prior to her appointment to BASICS Education Scotland over a year ago, she worked for the British Heart Foundation for eight years as Community Resuscitation Co-ordinator for Scotland, developing public and schools programmes for cardiopulmonary resuscitation (CPR) training, and advising and assessing public access defibrillation grants.

Debbie Danitsch
Consultant Nurse - Cardiothoracic Nursing
DHSc, MSc, BEd (Hons), DipN (Lond), PGDEA, RNT, RGN
Debbie has spent most of her nursing career caring for acutely/critically ill adults. She secured a consultant nurse role in cardiothoracics in 2002, at the time the first and only role nationally of its kind. She successfully finished her doctoral studies in 2009. She has vast experience working on cardiac advanced life support courses, developing protocols that have since been used by the European Resuscitation Council.

Sarah Dickie
Nurse Consultant - Emergency Nursing
MBA, PGC Teaching & Learning in Higher Education, PGCE Health Research, BSc (Hons) Nursing, RGN, ENB199
Sarah is a nurse consultant working in unscheduled care pan-Ayrshire for NHS Ayrshire & Arran, a joint appointment with the University of the West of Scotland. The major focus for her clinical expertise is in emergency care. She has previously worked as a research nurse on a critical care transfer project in Yorkshire and is an instructor on the Safe Transfer and Retrieval course (STaR).

Anne Dormer
BHF Lead Nurse Heart Failure
MSc, BSc (Hons), RN
Anne has worked to lead and deliver services for heart failure patients since 2001. Education is an important part of her role and she spent several years organising the North West Heart Failure Forum before handing over the

facilitation of this group to the Greater Manchester and Cheshire Cardiac Network in 2010. The forum delivers study days and networking opportunities for heart failure nurses and healthcare professionals with an interest in heart failure in the north west of England.

Fiona Foxall
Lecturer in Nursing
MA Medical Ethics, (BSc) Hons Nursing Studies, DPSN, PGCE(FAHE), ENB100, RN

Fiona Foxall qualified as a Registered General Nurse in 1984 and worked as a senior intensive care sister until 1990, when she moved into nurse education. She has always maintained clinical currency and competence by continuing to practise, teaching critical care nurses and undertaking continuing professional development within the intensive care setting. She was employed as the head of continuing development in the School of Health at the University of Wolverhampton but now lives and works in Australia.

Tim Grove
Exercise Specialist (Cardiac Rehabilitation Services)
MSc

Tim has been an exercise specialist in cardiac rehabilitation for nearly 10 years and he currently co-ordinates the exercise component of Heatherwood and Wexham Park hospitals phase III cardiac rehabilitation programme. He graduated in 2007 with a master's degree in cardiovascular rehabilitation from the University of Chester and he lectures and assesses on the British Association for Cardiac Rehabilitation's Phase IV Exercise Instructor course. Tim has also published in peer-reviewed journals, fitness magazines and presented poster presentations at the European Society of Cardiology's world congress and at the British Association for Cardiac Rehabilitation's conference.

Ian Jones
Senior Lecturer in Cardiac Nursing
RN, PhD

Ian qualified as a nurse in 1990 and has spent the past two decades working in cardiac care. He is a former president of the British Association for Nursing in Cardiovascular Care and has published widely in the field. He is currently employed as a senior lecturer in cardiac nursing and nurse researcher at the University of Salford in Greater Manchester.

Jan Keenan
Consultant Nurse - Cardiac Medicine
RGN, Nurse Prescriber, RNT, MSc Health Studies, PGD Higher Professional Education

Jan has been the consultant nurse in cardiac medicine at the Oxford Radcliffe Hospitals NHS Trust since 2001. She holds an Honorary Teaching Fellowship at the School of Health and Social Care, Oxford Brookes University. She is currently President and Honorary Secretary of the British Association of

Nurses in Cardiovascular Care and a council member of the British Cardiovascular Society. Jan holds a highly clinically focused role and works across the team to achieve demonstrable improvements across the patient pathway in the cardiac directorate at the ORH, as well as influencing the wider organisational and national agenda for nursing and cardiac care.

John McGowan
Senior Resuscitation Officer
RGN, RMN, MSc, BSc (Hons), BA, DIMC, RCSEd
John has been the resuscitation officer at the Southern General Hospital Glasgow since 1993. His special interests include acute cardiovascular care, resuscitation in childhood, environmental medicine and pre-hospital care.

Claire Rushton
Lecturer in Nursing
MA, BA (Hons), PGCHE, Dip Critical Care Nursing, DipN, RN (Adult)
Claire is a lecturer in the School of Nursing and Midwifery at Keele University. She contributes to teaching in foundation and adult branch pre-registration nursing courses at diploma and degree level. She also contributes to the Learning Beyond Registration teaching portfolio and takes the lead for the module on legal and ethical issues in healthcare. Her clinical background is in cardiology nursing. Her interests include end-of-life care and she has completed a MA in medical ethics and law through which she explored the potential impact of the Mental Capacity Act (2005) on women's end-of-life decision making. Claire is also interested in heart failure and co-morbidity, and particularly the impact of co-morbidity on changing prognosis in heart failure. She is a peer reviewer for the *British Journal of Cardiac Nursing*.

Pauline Walsh
Head of School, Nursing and Midwifery, Keele University
MA Medical Ethics & Law, DPSN, ENB100, RGN, ONC.
Pauline started her nursing career in Gloucestershire, qualifying in 1984, and worked clinically in trauma orthopaedics, surgery and intensive care nursing. Her academic interests revolve around healthcare ethics and professional practice, and she gained a master's degree in medical ethics in 1991 with a specific focus on life and death decision making. Since September 2010 she has been head of school in nursing and midwifery at Keele University.

Celia Warlow
Senior Resuscitation Officer
MA (Ed Man), BSc, Cert Ed, RGN
Celia is resuscitation services manager at Northampton General Hospital NHS Trust. She has worked in the field of resuscitation practice for 21 years, and is passionate about her role and improving all aspects of this field of science. Celia led a small team to develop an MSc in resuscitation practice at Brighton University in 2005, where she holds honorary lecturer status. She has also been an educational advisor to the Resuscitation Council (UK) since 1998.

Jackie Younker
Senior Lecturer in Nursing
BSN, MSN, PG CertEd
Jackie is currently a senior lecturer at the University of the West of England, Bristol. She has a background in cardiac and critical care nursing. She teaches clinical assessment skills and her areas of interest are advanced practice nursing, critical care and resuscitation.

Preface

The treatment of cardiac conditions has changed, and continues to change dramatically. The pace of change also appears to be accelerating. Cardiac conditions are common and life threatening, but thankfully there has never been a time where we have been able to do so much to lengthen and improve the lives of our patients. Specialist cardiac nurses form an elite cadre in healthcare and, as such, face many exciting challenges. Cardiac care probably involves more equipment and technology than any other field of medicine. Along with technology there are more drug treatments and an increasing role for nurses in prescribing and monitoring therapies. These times are without doubt the most exciting period in medical history in which to look after patients with cardiac disorders.

This book is designed to help the modern nurse tackle these challenges and to give new and experienced nurses an understanding of the key areas of cardiac disease. This knowledge can then be used to help patients with the understanding that this is a changing field: that what we have done in the past will give us experience and understanding, but that cardiac care is leading a healthcare revolution.

One of the key rewards of dealing with patients who are critically ill with cardiac conditions is that there are often dramatic improvements with modern treatments. The old-style Coronary Care Unit (CCU) of the 1970s and 1980s has changed beyond recognition, with most of the drama of the acute myocardial infarction (MI) being dealt with by primary percutaneous coronary intervention (PCI) in the cathlab. In that setting CCU can become a place where there are greater extremes of health. Some patients will feel completely well following their brief MI, which has been completely treated, immediately. The nurse looking after such patients may find the challenge will lie in getting cardiac rehabilitation messages on board in patients who can be so well and whose suffering was only relatively brief. The other end of the scale is that patients with major cardiac events are surviving for longer through the initial phase of illness and are having much more done for them acutely. Thus sicker, frailer and older patients may survive what were thought to be untreatable conditions. Their needs may be far more complex, both from a cardiological and nursing viewpoint.

Thus there are nursing care challenges because we are able to help people recover more quickly from very serious conditions and also because survival is better and patients are routinely offered more complex treatment.

Undoubtedly society's expectations of what can and should be delivered are also changing. Nursing has a key role in the interaction with the patient and family, which will have its own challenges.

Cardiac nurses are involved in the initial assessment and treatment of acute coronary syndromes (ACS) through to delivering definitive therapy, as well as aftercare and cardiac rehabilitation. Newer roles are now routine, such as helping to assess and monitor those patients whose ACS has been managed without intervention, and providing follow-up and secure hospital discharge. Nurse-led revascularisation clinics routinely provide follow-up for patients post PCI and coronary artery bypass graft (CABG). For those patients with significant risk of long-term serious ventricular arrhythmia, the nurse specialist can help guide them through the complexities of life-saving device therapy with implantable cardioverter defibrillators (ICD) and cardiac re-synchronisation therapy (CRT) implantation.

One of the greatest challenges is to provide a workforce with the necessary skills to deliver the care needed to meet these changing needs. The fundamentals and "anatomy" of the disease process are well understood. This book is a tool to cover the groundwork and encourage lifelong learning to meet the needs of such an exciting medical field. The professional rewards for being part of the cardiac healthcare team are being seen now.

Eighty to ninety percent of cardiology care in the UK is now delivered in the non-elective, urgent or emergency setting. This means that when patients attend with their first cardiac event they are being given "complete" treatment. Thus an ACS will often be the index event in a patient's complete inpatient revascularisation, arrhythmia management, etc. Therefore there is a need for nurses to understand all aspects of cardiac care when dealing with ACS patients as the patient's stay may encompass many cardiac treatments.

Dominic Cox
Consultant Editor

Acknowledgements

I would like to extend my sincere thanks to all of the contributing authors for their valuable contributions to this book; between them they have a wealth of clinical experience and expertise within the many and varied fields of cardiac care. I am particularly grateful to Rebecca McBride, who acted as a critical reader at many stages of the compilation process and offered much in the way of constructive feedback. I extend my thanks to the consultant editor, Dominic Cox, a great mentor and friend, for reviewing the clinical accuracy of the text and making helpful and valuable suggestions to improve it.

I would also like to thank the many undergraduate and postgraduate students I have worked with, in clinical practice and in the classroom, who have inspired me to find different ways of learning and teaching this amazingly dynamic and challenging subject area.

Melanie Humphreys

Chapter 1

Acute Coronary Syndrome in Perspective

Melanie Humphreys

Introduction

Significant change in how and where cardiac care is delivered has occurred since the National Service Framework (NSF) for Coronary Heart Disease (CHD) was first published in 2000. The pace of change has been rapid in terms of both clinical advances and different service models for delivery of care. Cardiac nurses now move seamlessly across organisational boundaries, moving from a patient's home, to the GP practice and acute trust setting (DH, 2005a).

Front-line clinicians and other practitioners continue to champion the development of cardiac services, bringing innovation and excellence to service development and delivery as practices and technologies evolve and advance.

Much of the content of the NSF for CHD is as relevant now as it was in 2000, and will probably still be relevant in 2020. As progress continues and the achievements that have already been realised are built upon, it is important that nurses continue to develop their own underpinning knowledge and enthusiasm to continue to grow within cardiac nursing. Patient expectation and need, technology and working practices in cardiology are continually advancing, and many nurses are in a position to contribute to the discussions about quality of care through the National Quality Board, which oversees the setting of priorities for the service in the future. Lord Darzi's report *High Quality Care For All* provided reaffirmation of the importance of putting quality at the centre of what all healthcare professionals do and the need to look across the whole patient pathway (DH, 2008a).

The challenge of saving lives

Cardiovascular disease is the UK's biggest cause of premature death and CHD accounts for more than 110,000 deaths in England each year. In March

2000, when the NSF for CHD was published, the chapters focused on CHD patient pathways; since then three important documents have been published. In March 2005, a final chapter was added on arrhythmia and sudden cardiac death. This focused on the care of patients living with dysrhythmias and families in which a sudden cardiac death had occurred (DH, 2005b). In May 2006, national commissioning guidance was published on the care of adolescents and adults with congenital heart disease (DH, 2006), and in 2008 a report on the National Infarct Angioplasty Project was published (DH, 2008b). This document sets out the new national strategy to treat heart attacks using primary angioplasty, which represents a major breakthrough in terms of reducing mortality, speed of rehabilitation and readmission rates. Many specialist cardiac nurses contributed to these important pieces of work, and many will continue to make positive contributions in the forthcoming years (DH, 2009a).

In *The Coronary Heart Disease National Service Framework, progress report for 2008* (DH, 2009a), the initial aims are discussed. These were to reduce mortality from heart disease and stroke and related circulatory diseases in people under 75 by at least 40% by 2010; this was set out in the public health White Paper *Saving Lives: Our Healthier Nation* in 1999. It was based on the trend data available at the time, including international comparisons, and was seen as a significant challenge. However, since then, steady progress has been made and the target has been met, five years ahead of schedule. This was considered to be a major achievement, attributable to the shared efforts of those working in many parts of the healthcare system. The report identified a number of specific achievements, including the following.

- People suffering a heart attack are receiving either:
  - thrombolysis, more quickly than before; or
  - primary angioplasty services.
- Waiting times for cardiac surgery have dropped dramatically since the publication of the NSF for CHD and outcomes have improved. In April 2002, there were 7,558 people waiting for a coronary artery bypass graft and 4,364 of them had been waiting three months or more; by December 2008 this had fallen to 1,670 people waiting and only six people had been waiting longer than three months (DH, 2009a).
- In primary care, secondary prevention has improved and is attributable to the additional incentive of the Quality and Outcomes Framework, a performance management system for GPs that is supervised by primary care trusts (PCTs) (DH, 2009b).
- The prescription rate for cholesterol-reducing statins has more than doubled over the past three years, cutting mortality from CHD and the number of heart attacks each year.
- Smoking cessation has also made a major contribution. Smoking prevalence among adults dropped from 28% in 1998 to 21% in 2007 (DH, 2009a).

Despite these examples of very positive trends within the realms of "saving lives", cardiovascular diseases (CVD) continue to exert a huge burden on individuals and society, with CHD remaining the single most common cause of death in the UK and other developed countries (British Heart Foundation, 2008), accounting for 198,000 deaths each year. One in three deaths (35%) is from CVD.The main forms of CVD are CHD and stroke. About half (48%) of all deaths from CVD are from CHD.

Coronary heart disease is the most common cause of death in the UK. Around one in five deaths in men and one in seven in women are from the disease (BHF, 2008). CHD causes around 94,000 deaths in the UK each year. Other forms of heart disease cause more than 31,000 deaths in the UK each year, so in total there were just under 126,000 deaths from heart disease in the UK in 2006.

Cardiovascular disease is one of the main causes of premature death in the UK (death before the age of 75). Thirty percent of premature deaths in men and 22% of premature deaths in women were from CVD in 2006 (BHF, 2008). CVD was responsible for more than 53,000 premature deaths in the UK in 2006.

Cardiovascular disease deaths as a whole have steadily declined since the 1970s, with a reported 27% reduction in mortality from heart disease, stroke and related diseases in people aged less than 75 years of age since 1996 (DH, 2005c).

Interestingly, UK morbidity data suggest that CHD prevalence is, in fact, increasing, and this seems to be particularly marked in people aged 75 years or more. A recent analysis by Majeed and Aylin (2005) suggests that by 2031:

- the number of cases of CHD will rise by 44% (to 3,190,000) and hospital admissions related to CHD will increase by 32% to 265,000
- the number of people with heart failure will rise by 54% (to 1,303,000) and hospital admissions will increase by 55% to 124,000
- the number of people with atrial fibrillation will rise by 46% (to 1,093,000) and hospital admissions will increase by 39% to 85,000.

While great progress has been made in moving cardiovascular care from tertiary prevention to secondary prevention, health plans must continue to drive CHD care further along the continuum towards primary prevention of CVD. CVD risk factors should be managed not only after a coronary event has occurred, but also before the onset of such an event. Ideally, healthy lifestyles should be promoted with all patients so that risk factors for CVD never develop. In this way, the future may well see CVD care moving from the inpatient setting to the outpatient setting.

The scope of this book

The acute coronary syndromes (ACS) represent the unstable phase of CHD and encompass a range of conditions that result in myocardial ischaemia or infarction. Despite advances in the knowledge of disease processes and improved pharmacological and interventional therapies, ACS continues to have significance for practitioners working across the spectrum of primary, secondary and tertiary care arenas (DH, 2009a).

Virtually every pathological process affecting the heart can lead to a critical cardiac event, and commonly sudden death within the community and within the hospital setting, therefore a good understanding of cardiac events and their immediate management is essential in optimising patient health and reducing mortality and morbidity. Through a structured approach of assessment, initiating investigations, treatment and delivering appropriate care, within the community and hospital setting, potentially life-threatening cardiac events can be identified. This will enable medical attention to be delivered in these situations, and ensure the most appropriate evidence-based care and treatment strategies are adopted (Humphreys, 2009).

Through a structured and focused approach this text offers a practical guide to nursing the cardiac patient; it addresses the management of cardiac patients within both community and hospital settings. It has relevance to nurses working across the nursing milieu, and will help to develop a comprehensive understanding of the contemporary evidence-based practice and principles underlying the care and management of the cardiac patient (Figure 1.1).

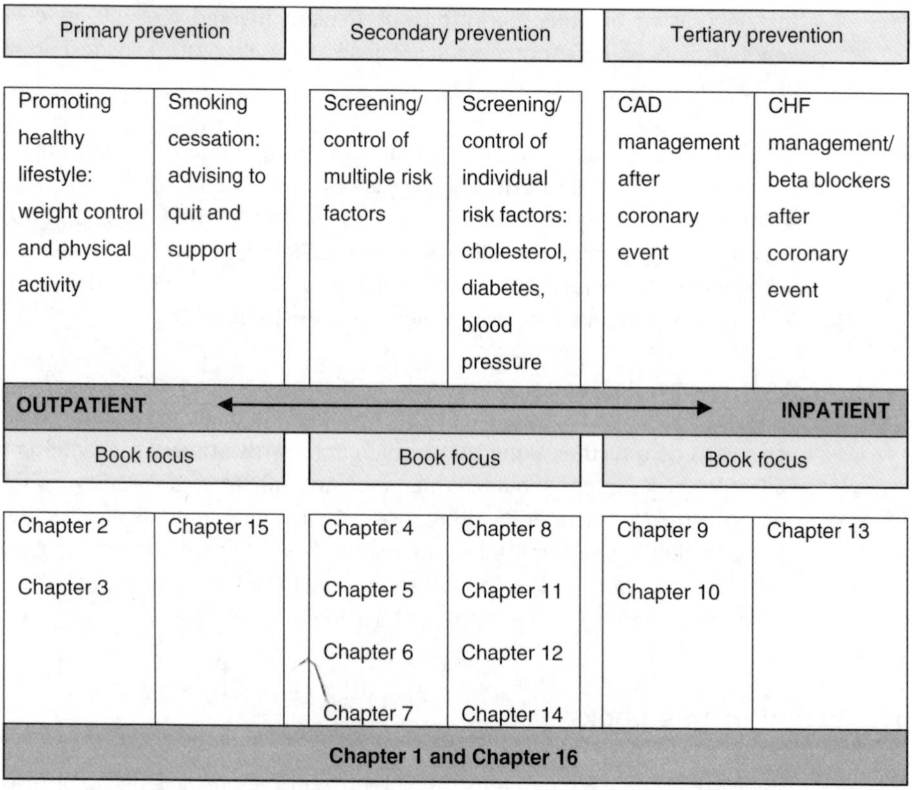

Primary prevention		Secondary prevention		Tertiary prevention	
Promoting healthy lifestyle: weight control and physical activity	Smoking cessation: advising to quit and support	Screening/ control of multiple risk factors	Screening/ control of individual risk factors: cholesterol, diabetes, blood pressure	CAD management after coronary event	CHF management/ beta blockers after coronary event
OUTPATIENT ←——————————————————————————→ **INPATIENT**					
Book focus		Book focus		Book focus	
Chapter 2 Chapter 3	Chapter 15	Chapter 4 Chapter 5 Chapter 6 Chapter 7	Chapter 8 Chapter 11 Chapter 12 Chapter 14	Chapter 9 Chapter 10	Chapter 13
Chapter 1 and Chapter 16					

Figure 1.1 The cardiovascular disease continuum.

As cardiac events have huge significance for all practitioners, this book will prove to be a practical resource for many nurses working within both general and specialist emergency/cardiac hospital settings. It will also have relevance for primary care workers wishing to develop their knowledge within all aspects of cardiac care, and as such will appeal to paramedics and other healthcare professionals working within general practice.

References

British Heart Foundation (BHF) (2008) Coronary heart disease statistics database. www.heartstats.org

Department of Health (2009a) *The Coronary Heart Disease National Service Framework: Building on Excellence, Maintaining Progress; progress report for 2008*. London, Department of Health.

Department of Health (2009b) *Developing the Quality and Outcomes Framework: Proposals for a New, Independent Process: Consultation Response and Analysis*. London, Department of Health.

Department of Health (2008a) *High Quality Care For All: NHS Next Stage Review final report*. London, Department of Health.

Department of Health (2008b) *National Infarct Angioplasty Project (NIAP) interim report*. London, Department of Health.

Department of Health (2006) *A Commissioning Guide for Services for Young People and Grown Ups with Congenital Heart Disease (GUCH)*. London, The Stationery Office.

Department of Health (2005a) *Creating a Patient-led NHS: Delivering the NHS Improvement Plan*. London, Department of Health.

Department of Health (2005b) Arrhythmias and sudden cardiac death. *National Service Framework for Coronary Heart Disease*. London, The Stationery Office.

Department of Health (2005c) *Leading the Way: The Coronary Heart Disease National Service Framework; progress report*. London, The Stationery Office.

Department of Health (2000) *National Service Framework for Coronary Heart Disease*. London, The Stationery Office.

Department of Health (1999) *Saving Lives: Our Healthier Nation*. London, The Stationery Office.

Humphreys M (2009) Cardiac emergencies. In: Jevon P, Humphreys M and Ewens B *Nursing Medical Emergency Patients*. Oxford, Blackwell Publishing.

Majeed A and Aylin P (2005) Dr Foster's case notes. The ageing population of the United Kingdom and cardiovascular disease. *British Medical Journal* **331**: 1362.

Chapter 2

Reducing the Risk: Primary Care Initiatives

Melanie Humphreys and Brenda Cottam

Introduction

Before the publication of the National Service Framework (NSF) for Coronary Heart Disease (CHD) (DH 2000a), the state of cardiovascular prevention and care in England was considered by many to be below the standard of other comparable Western countries. The UK as a whole had higher mortality and morbidity from coronary heart disease (CHD). Mortality was falling at a slower rate than elsewhere and there was clear evidence from published national and international studies that access to specialist care, including coronary revascularisation, was lower than in other countries (Quinn, 2007).

Coronary heart disease, stroke and related conditions remain a major cause of early death; however, mortality rates are reportedly falling due to improved treatment of cardiovascular events and improved management of primary preventative strategies, such as smoking cessation. In the UK, primary prevention treatment has produced three times the impact on mortality that secondary prevention management has (Kelly and Capewell, 2004). The prescription rate for cholesterol-reducing statins more than doubled from 2006 to 2009, cutting mortality from CHD and the number of heart attacks each year. Smoking cessation has also made a major contribution. Smoking prevalence among adults dropped from 28% in 1998 to 21% in 2007 (DH, 2009a). Secondary prevention has improved further within primary care, attributable to the additional incentive of the Quality and Outcomes Framework (DH, 2009b). The aim of this chapter is to understand the approach to primary care strategies aimed at reducing the risk of acute cardiac events.

Nursing the Cardiac Patient, First Edition. Edited by Melanie Humphreys.
© 2011 Blackwell Publishing Ltd. Published 2011 by Blackwell Publishing Ltd.

Learning outcomes

At the end of this chapter the reader will be able to:

- describe, using evidence-based sources, an overview of the referral and assessment process used within primary care
- critically discuss the importance of current rapid diagnostic clinics and investigations
- outline the significance of sudden cardiac death
- critically discuss the significance of community schemes and their impact within primary care.

Primary care initiatives in perspective

Saving Lives: Our Healthier Nation, published as a White Paper in July 1999 (DH, 1999), set a target to reduce the death rate from CHD and stroke and related diseases in people below the age of 75 by at least 40% by 2010. Following the launch of the NSF on 6 March 2000, CHD was firmly established as a priority area across government. The paper identified primary prevention as a crucial means of reducing prevalence of CHD. Standard four of the NSF for CHD states that "general practitioners and primary health care team should identify all people at significant risk of cardiovascular disease but who have not yet developed symptoms and offer them appropriate advice and treatment to reduce their risks" (p.4). Milestone three of Chapter 2 suggests that "every practice should have a protocol describing the systematic assessment, treatment and follow-up of people . . . whose risk of CHD events is >30% over ten years" (p.16), setting the way for a clear strategic direction for the management of CHD. The publication of the 10-year NHS plan (DH, 2000b) four months later reconfirmed key "immediate priority" milestones for delivery of the NSF, including the establishment of Rapid Access Chest Pain Clinics (RACPCs), increased revascularisation capacity and faster treatment, including, where necessary, pre-hospital thrombolysis delivered by paramedics. Smoking cessation was given high priority as a "key plank" of the wider public health programme; by 2004 at least a quarter of a million people had been helped to quit smoking for at least four weeks. A school fruit programme was instituted to ensure that around nine million children aged four to six years received at least one piece of fresh fruit every school day (Boyle, 2004).

The Health and Social Care Standards and Planning Framework 2005/6-2006/7 states that "in primary care, practice based registers [should be up-dated] so that patients with CHD and diabetes continue to receive appropriate advice and treatment in line with NSF standards and, by March 2006, ensure practice-based registers and systematic treatment regimes, including appropriate advice on diet, physical activity and smoking, also cover the majority of patients at high risk of CHD, particularly those with hypertension, diabetes and a BMI greater than 30" (DH, 2004). The Public Health White Paper *Choosing Health: Making Healthy Choices* sets outs the government's agenda to provide more opportunities, support and information for people who want to adopt a healthier lifestyle, which will contribute towards combating the modifiable risk factors that cause CHD (DH, 2005c).

Among the host of reforms since 1997, one of the most significant underpinning the NSF was arguably the renegotiation of the general medical services contract for general practitioners (GPs), which from April 2004 introduced a system of financial reward for performance on key areas including CHD in primary care (Quinn, 2007). A key component of the Quality and Outcomes Framework (QoF) was for improvements in patient care across four domains: clinical, organisational, "additional services" and patient experience. CVD, with diabetes and hypertension, forms a major component of the "points" attracting financial reward in the clinical domain. Use of disease registers in primary care, alongside improvements in clinical coding and protocols, also attract points under the organisational and patient experience domains (Capps, 2004). The QoF data have also been useful in providing epidemiological insights into the relationship between CHD prevalence, quality of care and socioeconomic deprivation (Strong *et al.*, 2006).

Identification of those "at risk"

The Framingham risk scoring system is widely used and available via many general practice computer systems to score each patient's relevant risk factors; these are then calculated to determine 10-year (short-term) risk for developing CHD (Grundy *et al.*, 2001). Framingham risks include:

- age
- sex
- HDL cholesterol
- total cholesterol
- systolic blood pressure
- smoking status
- diabetic status
- family history of ischaemic heart disease (IHD).
- electrocardiogram (ECG) evidence of left ventricular hypertrophy (optional).

However, not all practices use the Framingham software. The INTERHEART study lists nine categories that account for more than 90% of the associated risks of initial myocardial infarction (Yusuf *et al.*, 2004). Consistent results were found across 52 countries worldwide. They suggest that most premature myocardial infarction can be prevented if treatment is offered to the younger cohort of patients.

They conclude that worldwide, the two most important risk factors, which contribute to two-thirds of risk, are:

- smoking
- abnormal ratio of blood lipids.

Other important risk factors in men and women are:

- diabetes
- hypertension
- abdominal obesity
- psychosocial factors, i.e. stress
- lack of daily consumption of fruits and vegetables
- lack of daily exercise.

Modest alcohol consumption (three to four drinks weekly) has been determined to be a preventative measure (these factors are explored further in Chapters 14 and 15).

Collins and Altman (2009) have assessed the performance of the QRISK cardiovascular risk prediction algorithm in a primary care setting in the UK, and have compared QRISK with equivalent Framingham algorithms. The QRISK algorithm is based on the largest risk prediction study ever undertaken and highlights a potential use of large scale electronic health record systems. A team has linked electronic health records from several million people to produce a cardiovascular risk prediction algorithm that is claimed to be more accurate and better validated than previous ones. Although prediction algorithms are available for many conditions, most are based on small numbers, are poorly validated, infrequently updated and not generalisable. Moreover, most prediction algorithms are weak predictors and are not used regularly. QRISK is just the first of many continuously updatable prediction algorithms that will become available worldwide as electronic health record systems replace current paper-based systems. The planned UK General Practitioner Extraction Service, for example, should soon be capturing data relevant to risk prediction from most of the population (GPES, 2009). The sharing of such algorithms is considered to be the best way to facilitate their effective implementation (Jackson et al., 2009).

The NSF for CHD advises that patients who have a 10-year risk greater than 30% be added to the at-risk register and offered the same lifestyle advice and treatment as those patients already suffering with CHD, especially with a body mass index (BMI) >30. However, BMI as an indicator of risk has been challenged, with greater focus being placed on high-risk abdominally obese patients rather than BMI (Despres et al., 2001; Grundy et al., 2001), this was also identified in the INTERHEART study (Yusuf et al., 2004). Despres et al. (2001) state that the simple measurement of the waist circumference can indicate accumulation of abdominal fat; adding fasting triglyceride concentrations to the waist measurement would improve the practitioner's ability to identify abdominally obese men likely to have the features of the insulin resistance syndrome. This study focused on men, and there is little evidence to support this theory for women. This is an area where more research is needed.

Viscerally obese men are characterised by an atherogenic plasma lipoprotein profile.

- A triad of non-traditional markers for CHD found in viscerally obese middle-aged men (hyperinsulinaemia, raised apolipoprotein B concentration, and small LDL particles) increases the risk of CHD 20-fold.
- Even in the absence of hypercholesterolaemia, hyperglycaemia or hypertension, obese patients could be at high risk of CHD if they have this "hypertriglyceridaemic waist" phenotype.

The INTERHEART study claims that the effect of the nine risk factors are consistent in men and women, across different geographic regions and by ethnic group, making the study applicable worldwide. Among the implications of this study the concept of a uniform preventative strategy for heart attack across the world appears very attractive and of great potential impact. The ways in which the heart attacks that follow from the nine risk factors reflect the interplay of environmental and constitutional (genetic) influences remain to be further explored.

Rapid access chest pain clinics

Chest pain is a major burden on patients and the NHS, resulting in an estimated 634,000 primary care consultations (Stewart *et al.*, 2003). They make up a large proportion of emergency department (ED) attendances and acute medical admissions (Goodacre *et al.*, 2005), and many of these patients do indeed have an acute coronary syndrome (ACS). Stable angina pectoris is a common condition in the UK, with an estimated 96,000 new cases each year, and 955,000 people currently living with the condition (BHF, 2009). The incidence rises with age and is higher in men.

The NSF set out plans to establish rapid access chest pain clinics (RACPCs) throughout England in order that new patients with new onset chest pain, referred by their GP, could undergo timely specialist assessment (DH, 2000a). Referral to an RACPC is facilitated by protocols agreed at the primary/secondary care interface supported by the local cardiac network. Standardised pro formas are widely used to ensure appropriate use of the RACPC for its intended purpose (the RACPC is not appropriate for patients with suspected ACS or those with known CHD already under the care of the cardiology department) and to minimise delay (Quinn, 2007). The RACPC specialist nurse undertakes baseline history and clinical examination. A normal ECG does not rule out CHD but provides a baseline and helps to exclude factors such as bundle branch block, which would hamper analysis of an exercise test. If the clinical picture suggests new onset stable angina, an exercise tolerance test is usually performed. Additional tests considered would include:

- stress echocardiography
- myocardial perfusion imaging
- magnetic resonance imaging (MRI)
- cardiac computer tomography (CT)
- calcium scoring.

Studies have suggested that the RACPC has provided an efficient and effective substitution for the traditional cardiology outpatient clinic model (Smallwood, 2009; Taylor *et al.*, 2008; Sekhri *et al.*, 2006). The establishment of RACPCs in England demanded many new skills from nurses working in cardiac care to ensure that competent cardiac assessment and management is facilitated. The focus of these clinics remains to provide a high level of care and assessment to patients admitted with chest pain or a cardiac arrhythmia. Practitioners working in RACPCs have developed their roles and often offer chest pain assessment services throughout acute and emergency care areas (Smallwood, 2009). Such advanced roles are established to augment, rather than replace, the doctor's role (DH, 2005a). Many working in chest pain assessment teams were involved in meeting the thrombolysis targets through nurse-initiated thrombolysis; the emphasis has now focused on timely referral for primary angioplasty (DH, 2009).

Other roles and skills these practitioners may develop and offer include:

- 24-hour cardiac assessment
- stratification of patients according to risk
- initiating treatment strategies for ACS
- prescribing
- interpretation of heart and lung sounds
- advanced interpretation of ECGs
- advanced life support skills
- teaching
- offering advice and support to junior doctors and nurses
- diagnosis and treatment of arrhythmias
- managing nurse-led clinics
- liaising with senior medics to request and interpret relevant tests, i.e. exercise tests, angiograms
- follow-up clinics for patients post revascularisation and for medically managed patients with ACS.

The Healthcare Commission undertook a formal evaluation of NSF implementation in 2005 (Healthcare Commission, 2005), reporting evidence of significant progress towards many of the national standards, particularly in relation to heart attack treatment, faster diagnosis of angina and reducing waits for revascularisation, underpinned by increased investment and targeted modernisation initiatives. The commission report also recognised the significant advances made in development of primary care CHD registers, but highlighted the need for further work to improve preventive work on a population basis and to provide better care for patients with heart failure or requiring cardiac rehabilitation (these will be explored within Chapters 13, 14 and 15).

The delivery of community-based services continues to be developed; the White Paper *Our Health, Our Care, Our Say: A New Direction For Community Services* (Secretary of State for Health, 2006) sets out a vision for health and social care delivered outside hospitals, identifying five areas for change.

- Improved access and more funding following the patient, ensuring personalised care, and expansion of walk-in (health) centres in the community.
- The shifting of care away from hospitals closer to people's homes, and investment in community hospitals and facilities.
- Improving working and information sharing between health and social care, and better co-ordination between the NHS and local councils.
- Budgets to increase choice by direct payment or care budget for people to pay for their own home help or care. PCTs required to act on findings of patient surveys.
- More action on prevention through introduction of the NHS "life check" at key points in an individual's life, and linking the London 2012 Olympics to a "Fitter Britain" campaign (Secretary of State for Health, 2006).

The implications of these reforms for services for patients with chest pain are unclear, but it is possible that chest pain assessment clinics and similar services could be situated in diagnostic centres run by GPs (DH, 2009; DH, 2008; DH, 2005b).

Sudden cardiac death

Sudden cardiac death is still the most important cause of premature death in the industrialised world, accounting for 700,000 deaths per year in Europe (Handley *et al.*, 2005; Priori *et al.*, 2004); with CHD remaining the UK's biggest killer. In the European guidelines for resuscitation published in 2005, Handley *et al.* state that some 40% of victims suffering sudden cardiac arrest are known to be in ventricular fibrillation (VF) or pulseless ventricular tachycardia (VT), and postulate that this figure is likely to be much higher, but this remains unknown as it is not monitored in the first few minutes after cardiac arrest.

Early recognition and access to emergency services

Mueller *et al.* (2006) contest that "sudden" cardiac death is not always just that. Indeed, signs and symptoms are evident for some time before cardiac arrest occurs, thus meaning this could be a very preventable cause of death if public education about recognising warning signs truly reached its target. They also contend that although early cardiopulmonary resuscitation (CPR) and early defibrillation undeniably saves lives, where this is targeted (e.g. public places) could be misdirected, as most deaths occur in the home or a residential area, where bystander CPR and access to defibrillation is least likely. Advertising campaigns supporting the recognition of the symptoms of ACS have been targeted to raise public awareness and the emphasis on the need to make early 999 calls.

Early CPR

Eisenburger and Safar (1999) report the value of early CPR, which has been well established. They remind us that the impact of bystander CPR (BCPR) is well documented, showing that the increase in survival from cardiac arrest can be doubled in areas where extensive public CPR programmes operate.

Community CPR and first aid training is now commonly accessible in most areas throughout the UK via:

- first aid training agencies
- voluntary aid societies
- public access by voluntary groups
- workplaces, through first aid at work.

In the UK, statutory NHS ambulance services aim to reach 75% of cardiac arrest and chest pain (and other immediately life-threatening) emergency calls within a nationally set target time of eight minutes (measured under "call connect"). However, within three to four minutes post-arrest, cerebral damage becomes a significant factor (Eisenburger and Safar, 1999). Therefore survival from cardiac arrest depends on:

- early recognition and call to emergency services
- early CPR to reverse the effects of hypoxia
- early defibrillation to correct VF or VT, both associated with sudden cardiac arrest.

This is now well established in the discipline of resuscitation, and the Chain of Survival first conceptualised by Cummins et al. in 1991 (in Handley et al., 2005) is now the mantra of modern-day resuscitation (Figure 2.1).

This means that bystander and community-based CPR plays a significant role in return of spontaneous circulation (ROSC) after cardiac arrest. However, audits of out of hospital cardiac arrest still show the frequency of BCPR remains poor, with less than one-third of cardiac arrest victims benefiting from BCPR before emergency services arrive (Eisenburger and Safar, 1999). The importance of BCPR is evidenced in one UK study by Dowie et al.

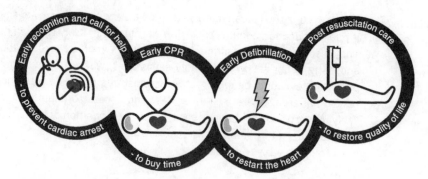

Figure 2.1 The Chain of Survival. Reproduced with permission from Laerdal Medical Ltd.

(2003). Their work with the London Ambulance Service showed that BCPR increased the chance of survival by 10% over a monitored period of time. However, this study demonstrated a high percentage of BCPR (44%) in progress when the ambulance arrived.

Early defibrillation

In the past few decades, the advent of automated external defibrillators (AEDs) in public places has meant that early access to defibrillation has become much more common. Advances in manufacturing and technology mean these simple and accurate AEDs can be used safely in workplaces, public places and even in the home (Jorgensen et al., 2003). Evidence is undisputed regarding the significance of early defibrillation. When the International Liaison Committee on Resuscitation (ILCOR) published its guidelines for CPR and emergency cardiac care in 2000, it stated:

> With reported survival rates of up to 49%, PAD (public access defibrillation) has the potential to be the single greatest advance in the treatment of prehospital sudden cardiac death since the invention of CPR.

Yet appropriate placement of AEDs is still contested. Handley et al. (2005) reflect the most common opinion that defibrillators should be sited in places where large numbers of the public gather or pass though (railway stations, airports, shopping centres etc) and where cardiac arrests occur once every two years or more. Similarly, remote areas where ambulance response times are likely to be extended also influence where AEDs and community based programmes should be sited. This is supported by most national defibrillation programme planners and ILCOR (2000) suggest that PAD programmes prove to be cost effective when measured against years of added life. However, Handley et al (2005) remind us that up to 80% of cardiac arrests occur in residential or private settings. This then needs to be addressed through emergency dispatch systems to enable rapid responses with a defibrillator to residential settings as well as public places. Community first responders must therefore arrive on scene within five minutes – before emergency medical services – to be a truly effective resource, although their target response time is eight minutes.

The European Resuscitation Council and the European Society of Cardiology recognised the significance of community-based defibrillation and in 2004 produced policy statements making recommendations surrounding the use of AEDs in Europe. These included guidance for:

- legislation
- training and updating lay and co-responders
- access to and via emergency service call systems
- audit of AED use
- needs analyses
- cost benefits to public health.

First responders

The UK has seen rapid development of first and community first responder schemes in the last decade. Community first responders are:

> ... volunteers who respond to emergency calls within their local community. They are generally lay people who have received basic medical training from their ambulance service. They respond, when available, to immediately life-threatening calls, usually in a rural area or one that is difficult for ambulances to reach within the current time target of eight minutes. They are not a substitute for professional paramedics and technicians, but they augment the ambulance service's response.
>
> (Healthcare Commission, 2007)

First responders come from a variety of backgrounds – from co-responders in other emergency services (police, fire, coastguard), staff in public places providing a localised emergency response (e.g. shopping centres, railway stations and airports), first aid organisation partners or volunteers from military backgrounds, to the general public keen to support emergency response systems in their local communities. They are not employees of ambulance services, but when called out by the ambulance services act as agents for them as part of the emergency response (Healthcare Commission 2007). Many nurses and healthcare practitioners are taking up this voluntary role.

First responder groups are set up in areas of identified need – now mostly influenced and defined by local ambulance service audit data in order to be sure of a co-ordinated response backed up by technicians/paramedics. The Healthcare Commission (2007) indicated that ambulance services see benefits in community first responder schemes, which have already had a positive impact on response times.

Colquhoun *et al.* (2008) show that although community first responders attending home and community-based cardiac arrests is a relatively new concept in the UK, and cost benefits have not yet been evaluated, they are worthy of support and continued funding to prove their value in time. They showed that these responders are achieving comparable results to the ambulance services. The key to ongoing work is that any public access and community response defibrillation programme must be aligned to the ambulance services based on data about incidence of sudden cardiac arrest and response times (Priori *et al.*, 2004).

Summary

Coronary heart disease continues to exert a huge burden on patients, families, health services and society. Chest pain and sudden death form major parts of that burden. Implementation of the NSF has been associated with many improvements in care, including faster access to care and uptake of evidence-based treatments in both primary and secondary care settings. Preventative strategies have continued to have a high national profile. As the NHS undergoes significant reorganisation and care becomes more community focused, cardiac nurses will need to continue to develop their skills and expertise towards working in these challenging times, in order to contribute to reducing the cardiac risk.

References

Boyle R (2004) Meeting the challenge of cardiovascular care in the new National Health Service. *Heart* **90** (suppl. IV): iv3-iv5.

British Heart Foundation (BHF) (2009) Coronary heart disease statistics database. www.heartstats.org

Capps N (2004) Quality and outcomes framework of the new general medical services contract. Guest editorial. National Electronic Library for Health. Cardiovascular Diseases Specialist Library. www.library.nhs.uk/CARDIOVASCULAR/Page.aspx?pagename=GUESTARC

Collins GS and Altman DG (2009) An independent external validation and evaluation of QRISK cardiovascular risk prediction: a prospective open cohort study. *British Medical Journal* **339**: b2584. www.bmj.com/cgi/content/abstract/339/jul07_2/b2584

Colquhoun MC, Chamberlain DA, Newcombe RG *et al.* (2008) A national scheme for public access defibrillation in England and Wales: early results. *Resuscitation* **78**: 275-80.

Commission for Healthcare Audit and Inspection (Healthcare Commission) (2007) *The Role and Management of Community First Responders. Findings from a national survey of NHS ambulance services in England.* London, Healthcare Commission.

Department of Health (2009a) *The Coronary Heart Disease National Service Framework: Building on Excellence, Maintaining Progress; progress report for 2008*. London, Department of Health.

Department of Health (2009b) *Developing the Quality and Outcomes Framework: Proposals for a New, Independent Process; consultation response and analysis*. London, Department of Health.

Department of Health (2008) *High Quality Care For All: NHS Next Stage Review final report*. London, Department of Health.

Department of Health (2005a) Arrhythmias and sudden cardiac death. *National Service Framework for Coronary Heart Disease*. London, The Stationery Office.

Department of Health (2005b) *Creating a Patient-led NHS: Delivering the NHS Improvement Plan*. London, Department of Health.

Department of Health (2005c) *Leading the Way: the Coronary Heart Disease National Service Framework; progress report*. London, The Stationery Office.

Department of Health (2004) *National Standards, Local Action: Health and Social Care Standards and Planning Framework 2005/06-2007/08*. London, Department of Health.

Department of Health (2000a) *National Service Framework for Coronary Heart Disease*. London, The Stationery Office.

Department of Health (2000b) *The NHS Plan*. London, The Stationery Office.

Department of Health (1999) *Saving Lives: Our Healthier Nation*. London, The Stationery Office.

Despres J-P, Lemieux I and Prud'homme D (2001) Treatment of obesity: need to focus on high risk abdominally obese patients. *British Medical Journal* **322**: 716.

Dowie R, Campbell H, Donohoe R and Clarke P (2003) "Event tree" analysis of out-of-hospital cardiac arrest data: confirming the importance of bystander CPR. *Resuscitation* **56**: 173-81.

Eisenburger P and Safar P (1999) Life supporting first aid training of the public – review and recommendations. *Resuscitation* **41**: 3-18.

General Practice Extraction Service (GPES) (2009) NHS Information Centre. www.ic.nhs.uk/services/in-development/general-practice-extraction-service

Goodacre S, Cross E, Arnold J, Angelini K, Capewell S and Nicholl J (2005) The health care burden of acute chest pain. *Heart* **91**: 229-30.

Grundy S, Cleeman J, Bairey Merz C *et al.* (2001) Implications of recent clinical trials for the national cholesterol education program adult treatment panel III guidelines. *Journal of the American College of Cardiology* **44**(3): 720-32.

Handley AJ, Koster R, Monsieurs K, Perkins GD, Davies S and Bossaert L (2005) European Resuscitation Council Guidelines for Resuscitation 2005. Section 2. Adult basic life support and use of automated external defibrillators. *Resuscitation* **67**(S1): S7-S23.

Healthcare Commission (2005) Getting To the Heart of It. Coronary Heart Disease in England: a review of progress towards national standards. London, Healthcare Commission. Available at: www.healthcarecommission.org.uk

International Liaison Committee on Resuscitation (2000) Guidelines 2000 for Cardiopulmonary Resuscitation and Emergency Cardiovascular Care. International consensus on science. *Supplement to Circulation* **102**(8): I4-I5.

Jackson R, Marshall R, Kerr A, Riddell T and Wells S (2009) QRISK or Framingham for predicting cardiovascular risk? *British Medical Journal* **339**: b2673. hwww.bmj.com/cgi/content/full/339/jul07_2/b2673#REF12#REF12

Jorgenson DB, Skarr T, Russell JK, Snyder DE and Uhrbrock K (2003) AED use in businesses, public facilities and homes by minimally trained first responders. *Resuscitation* **59**: 225-33.

Kelly MP and Capewell S (2004) *Relative Contributions of Changes in Risk Factors and Treatment to the Reduction in Coronary Heart Disease Mortality*. NHS, Health Development Agency. Available at: www.nice.org.uk/niceMedia/documents/CHD_Briefing_nov_04.pdf

Mueller D, Agrawal R and Arntz H-R (2006) How sudden is sudden cardiac death? *Resuscitation* **69**(1): 42.

Priori SG, Bossaert LL, Chamberlain DA *et al.* (2004) Policy statement ESC-ERC recommendations for the use of automated external defibrillators (AEDs) in Europe. *Resuscitation* **60**: 245–52.

Quinn T (2007) Coronary heart disease, healthcare policy and evolution of chest pain assessment and management in the UK. In: Albarran J and Tagney J *Chest Pain*. Oxford, Blackwell Publishing.

Secretary of State for Health (2006) *Our Health, Our Care, Our Say: A New Direction for Community Services*. Command Paper 6737. London, The Stationery Office.

Sekhri N, Feder GS, Junghans C, Hemingway H and Timmis AD (2006) Rapid access chest pain clinics and the traditional cardiology outpatient clinic. *Quarterly Journal of Medicine* **99**(3): 135–41.

Smallwood A (2009) Cardiac assessment teams: a focused ethnography of nurses' roles. *British Journal of Cardiac Nursing* **4**(3): 132–9.

Stewart S, Murphy N and Walker A (2003) The current cost of angina pectoris to the National Health Service in the UK. *Heart* **89**: 848–53.

Strong M, Maheswaran R and Radford J (2006) Socioeconomic deprivation, coronary heart disease prevalence and quality of care: a practice-level analysis in Rotherham using data from the new UK general practitioner Quality and Outcomes Framework. *Journal of Public Health* **28**(1): 39–42.

Taylor G, Murphy NF, Berry C *et al.* (2008) Long-term outcome of low-risk patients attending a rapid-assessment chest pain clinic. *Heart* **94**: 628–32

Yusuf S, Hawken S, Ôunpuu S *et al.* (2004) Effect of potentially modifiable risk factors associated with myocardial infarction in 52 countries (the INTERHEART study): case-control study. *Lancet* **364**(9438): 937–52.

Chapter 3

Assessment of the Cardiovascular System

Jackie Younker

Introduction

Assessment of the cardiovascular system is an essential skill when considering patients with cardiac disease. A thorough history and clinical examination will help the practitioner to make an insightful diagnosis for any number of presenting symptoms, the most common being chest pain. The assessment process begins by taking the patient's history. Subjective information from the history will provide insight into actual and potential problems and help to guide the physical examination further. The cardiovascular system examination findings, along with results of investigations, support or refute the differential diagnoses for patients who present with cardiovascular symptoms. Symptoms that often occur in heart disease include chest pain, palpitations, shortness of breath, fatigue, peripheral oedema and syncope (Kumar and Clark, 2005).

This chapter provides an overview of clinical examination skills used in assessment of the cardiovascular system. General techniques of inspection, palpation, percussion and auscultation will be used to describe the examination. The chapter also reviews assessment of the patient with chest pain, and key diagnostic procedures useful for assessing the cardiovascular system will be highlighted.

> ### Learning outcomes
>
> At the end of this chapter the reader will be able to:
>
> - describe the sequence used to examine the cardiovascular and peripheral vascular systems
> - recognise normal and common abnormal findings of the cardiovascular assessment
> - discuss assessment of the patient presenting with chest pain
> - consider electrocardiography, laboratory testing and diagnostic procedures as part of the cardiovascular assessment.

Nursing the Cardiac Patient, First Edition. Edited by Melanie Humphreys.
© 2011 Blackwell Publishing Ltd. Published 2011 by Blackwell Publishing Ltd.

Cardiovascular assessment in perspective

It is important for the patient and examiner to be appropriately prepared for the examination. Consideration must be given to providing a suitable environment, paying particular attention to privacy and dignity, lighting and temperature. Handwashing is essential before and on completion of the assessment. Equipment such as a stethoscope, blood pressure cuff and penlight should be readily available.

Examination of the cardiovascular system includes assessing heart function and arterial and venous circulation. The cardiovascular examination must be performed in a systematic way that is comfortable for both the patient and the examiner, and includes inspection, palpation and auscultation. The cardiovascular examination is generally done with the examiner on the patient's right side. Advantages of this position include:

- palpation of the apical impulse is more comfortable
- jugular venous pressure is better estimated from the right side (Bickley and Szilagyi, 2008).

The patient should be supine with the head of bed elevated to 30° to 45° for most of the examination. The patient may also need to turn on the left side and sit upright (Seidel *et al.*, 2003).

General examination

The patient's general wellbeing should be observed at the beginning of the examination. Looking at the patient's general presentation, height and weight, colour, facial expression, posture and gait at the beginning of the patient encounter helps to provide a picture of their general state of health. Specific findings such as obesity, cachexia, jaundice or pallor may be signs of cardiac disease that need further examination (Kumar and Clark, 2005). Other areas to observe include the following.

- Signs of shortness of breath, distress or use of accessory muscles – the normal respiratory rate is approximately 10–20 breaths/minute. Tachypnoea is a sign of heart disease, most commonly left ventricular failure (LVF). Oedema of the alveoli in the lungs will impair breathing and the respiratory effort will be increased to try to ventilate the lungs (Kumar and Clark, 2005). A respiratory examination may also be necessary if any altered respiratory findings are noted.
- Eyes, mouth and face:
  - colour, expression, sweating, pallor
  - mouth, lips and tongue for pallor, blue or grey colour, indicating central cyanosis and poor perfusion. This may occur when capillary oxygen saturation is less than 85% (Kumar and Clark, 2005). Patients with central cyanosis will also have peripheral cyanosis

- eyes for xanthelasma - irregularly shaped, yellow-tinted lipid deposits on periorbital tissue suggestive of hyperlipidaemia, these present as solid elevations of the skin
- periphery of the cornea for arcus - this presents as a grey ring around the iris and is indicative of precipitation of cholesterol crystals, which is suggestive of a high cholesterol level
- head and neck for symptoms of thyroid disease (hypothyroidism - dry, thin, coarse hair; hyperthyroidism - exophthalmos, goitre). Hypothyroidism or hyperthyroidism may cause arrhythmias, hypertension or heart failure.

- Upper extremities:
  - colour and temperature of hands and fingers - peripheral cyanosis may be due to cold. It also occurs in diseases associated with peripheral vasoconstriction and poor venous circulation
  - capillary refill time (CRT) - a prolonged CRT >2 seconds may indicate poor peripheral perfusion (Moule and Albarran, 2009)
  - fingernail clubbing suggests cyanotic heart disease or respiratory disease. The most common cardiac cause is congenital heart disease (Kumar and Clark, 2005).
  - splinter haemorrhages under the nails - these frequently occur due to trauma, but may indicate microembolism in endocarditis or other vascular conditions (Longmore et al., 2007).

- Lower extremities:
  - examination of the venous system in the lower limbs should always be undertaken. Expose the patient's legs
  - note the colour and temperature of legs and feet - blue, pale or mottled indicates poor arterial and/or venous circulation
  - note the size, symmetry and any presence of oedema - heart failure causes activation of the renin-angiotensin-aldosterone system, which leads to dependent oedema (Guyton and Hall, 2000). A deep vein thrombosis (DVT) may present with unilateral leg swelling (Bickley and Szilagyi, 2008).
  - observe the hair distribution - hair loss occurs with arterial insufficiency (Seidel et al., 2003)
  - venous pattern - signs of varicose veins. The veins will appear dilated and tortuous and the vessel walls may feel somewhat thickened (Bickley and Szilagyi, 2008).

Arterial pulses

Palpate radial pulses for rate, rhythm, quality and equality by compressing an artery against a bone. Typically, the right radial pulse is assessed first and used for comparison, findings may include:

- regular rhythm - sinus rhythm
- variation on breathing (usually quickening on inspiration) - sinus arrhythmia, this is a normal rhythm

- tachycardia >100 beats/minute
- bradycardia <50 beats/minute
- regularly irregular = type 1 – second degree heart block or coupled extra-systoles (pulsus bigeminus)
- irregularly irregular = atrial fibrillation, ventricular ectopic beats
- bounding = exercise, anxiety, fever/sepsis
- weak, difficult to palpate = low cardiac output
- inequality between left- and right-sided pulses = impaired circulation
- compare the apex beat with the radial pulse and check for a pulse deficit – in atrial fibrillation the heart rate is sometimes faster than the pulse, the difference being termed *pulse deficit*
- regularly irregular = type 1 – second degree heart block or coupled extra-systoles (pulsus bigeminus)
- irregularly irregular = atrial fibrillation, ventricular ectopic beats; these last two findings would be supported by electrocardiogram (ECG) presentation.

Blood pressure

Blood pressure should be measured in both arms. Systolic blood pressure may normally vary up to 10 mm Hg between the right and left arms. A variable pulse from atrial fibrillation may make a precise reading difficult. A difference of >20 mm Hg systolic between arms suggests arterial occlusion on the side with the lower pressure (Cox, 2004). Orthostatic (postural) hypotension is likely if there is a fall in systolic blood pressure of 20 mm Hg or more when the patient stands. Patients with an acute aortic dissection may present with an inter-arm blood pressure difference of >20 mm Hg. These patients most likely have accompanying symptoms such as chest pain, hypotension and neurologic changes (Kumar and Clark, 2005).

Jugular venous pressure (JVP)

Observing the internal jugular vein provides an estimation of right atrial pressure (Figure 3.1).

- Position the patient supine to fill the jugular veins.
- Gradually raise the head of the bed to approximately 45°. Look for jugular venous pulsations between the angle of the jaw and clavicle. It may be helpful to shine a torch at an angle across the neck. Venous pulsations are not usually palpable.
- Measure the vertical distance between the manubriosternal angle and the top of the venous column (point to where the vein is filled with blood). It may be helpful to place a ruler on the patient's chest and draw an imaginary line from the jugular pulsation to the ruler to estimate pressure.
- Normal JVP is usually <3 cm H_2O. This equates to an approximate right atrial pressure of 8 cm H_2O (Seidel *et al.*, 2005).

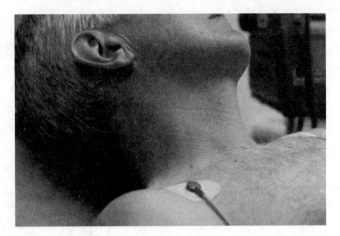

Figure 3.1 Patient position for estimating the JVP – the right jugular vein is clearly seen.

- A very low JVP cannot be measured this way and is likely caused by hypovolaemia due to haemorrhage.
- Jugular venous pressure is elevated in heart failure. Severe right heart failure, tricuspid insufficiency, constrictive pericarditis and cardiac tamponade may cause extreme elevation of JVP.
- Obesity makes it difficult to see the jugular vein pulsations.

Carotid pulse

The carotid pulse is not normally visible when looking at the neck. It can be palpated medial to and below the angle of the jaw. It is important not to palpate both sides simultaneously; this may decrease blood flow to the brain and cause the patient to have syncope (Bickley and Szilagyi, 2008). Listen over both carotid arteries with the stethoscope for the presence of bruits, a murmur-like or "whooshing" sound caused by constriction or altered flow. Ask the patient to hold a breath for a few seconds to make listening easier.

Examination of the precordium

Inspection, palpation and auscultation are used to examine the precordium (Figure 3.2). The exam is usually done with the patient at 30°. Other positions needed are turning to the left side and sitting upright.

Inspection
- Look at the precordium for deformities of the chest wall such as pectus excavatum (a depression in the lower part of the sternum) or kyphoscoliosis (an abnormal curvature of the spine) which may lead to compression of large vessels and cause an ejection systolic murmur (Kumar and Clark, 2005), also note any visible scars (sternotomy, lateral thoracotomy).

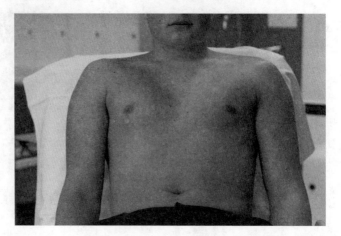

Figure 3.2 Exposure of the precordium, prior to inspection, palpation and auscultation.

- The apical impulse may be visible at approximately the midclavicular line, 5th intercostal space and is best observed when the patient is sitting up and the heart is closer to the chest wall. This is easily obscured by obesity, large breasts or a muscular chest, and doesn't necessarily present an abnormal finding.
- A readily visible and bounding apical impulse suggests a large left ventricle.
- Right ventricular hypertrophy or atrial enlargement may cause a heave over the left parasternal area.

Palpation
- Palpate the apical beat or point of maximal impulse (PMI). This is usual at 5th intercostal space, midclavicular line in adults. It may shift slightly to the 6th intercostal space, just left of the midclavicular line in older adults – its radius is usually no more than 1cm
- Ask the patient to lean forward or lay on the left side if the PMI is difficult to find. Apical impulses are usually impalpable in emphysema, obesity and effusions (pericardial or pleural)
- Assess the character of the impulse:
  - more vigorous than expected is described as a *heave* or *lift*
  - forceful or widely distributed – may indicate increased cardiac output or ventricular hypertrophy
  - thrusting displaced apical beat – suggests volume overload, possibly from mitral or aortic valve incompetence, left-to-right shunt, or cardiomyopathy
  - tapping apex beat – occurs in mitral stenosis.
- Palpate the left sternal border and the base. A palpable murmur that feels like a fine, rushing vibration is described as a *thrill*.

Auscultation

- The key is to use a systematic approach listening and describing what is heard. There are four valves (mitral, tricuspid, pulmonary and aortic) and each has an auscultatory area. These areas reflect sounds transmitted in the direction of blood flow as it passes through the valves, not surface markings of the valves. For this reason, there are five key listening areas:
  - aortic valve area - 2nd right intercostal space, right sternal border
  - pulmonary valve area - 2nd left intercostal space, left sternal border
  - second pulmonic area (Erb's point) - 3rd intercostal space, left sternal border
  - tricuspid area - 4th left intercostal space, lower left sternal border
  - mitral (apical) area - apex of the heart, 5th left intercostal space, mid-clavicular line.
- It is useful to listen over each main area with the bell and diaphragm of the stethoscope. The diaphragm is able to pick up relatively high-pitched sounds (S_1, S_2) while the bell transmits softer and lower pitched sounds (S_3, S_4, mitral stenosis murmur). Listen with the patient supine and sitting up, leaning slightly forward. Take time to listen carefully for each heart sound, isolating each component of the cardiac cycle. It may be helpful to palpate the carotid pulse to assist in determining systole and diastole, particularly when an irregular rhythm such as atrial fibrillation is present. Note any added sounds then listen for murmurs (Bickley and Szilagyi, 2008).
- Heart sounds are described by pitch, intensity, duration and timing in the cardiac cycle. Sounds produced are generally low pitched. S_1 and S_2 result from valve closure and are the most distinct sounds and provide useful clues about heart function:
  - **S_1** - mitral and tricuspid valve closure, indicates the beginning of systole, best heard towards the apex
  - **S_2** - aortic and pulmonic valve closure, indicates the end of systole, best heard in aortic and pulmonic areas, higher-pitched and shorter than S_1
  - **splitting of S_2** - S_2 is made up of two sounds that merge during expiration. Aortic valve closure (A_2) contributes most of the S_2 sound when heard in the aortic and pulmonic areas and tends to override the sound from pulmonic valve closure (P_2). During inspiration, P_2 occurs a little later and gives S_2 two phases or a split S_2. Listening while asking the patient to take a deep breath may reveal a split S_2. Normal or physiological splitting is common in children and young adults. In older adults a delayed closure of P_2 may be associated with right ventricular hypertrophy or pulmonary hypertension
  - **S_3** - first phase of rapid ventricular filling in early diastole; increased with exercise, fast heart rate, elevation of legs and increased venous return. Often described as a ventricular gallop and heard best at the apex

- S_4 - second phase of ventricular filling; atrial contraction causing ventricular filling towards the end of diastole, heard just before S_1. A physiological S_4 may be heard in middle-aged adults, particularly after exercise. In older adults suspect hypertensive disease, coronary artery disease, myocardial ischaemia, infarction or congestive heart failure. Often described as an atrial gallop.

- Extra heart sounds - heart valves usually open without making a noise unless thickened or roughened. Extra heart sounds are described as:
  - *ejection clicks* are heard when deformed but mobile aortic or pulmonic valves open. This sound is heard early in systole
  - *opening snaps* are associated with an abnormal mitral or tricuspid valve and are best heard in diastole
  - a *pericardial friction rub* may be heard when inflammation of the pericardial sac causes the parietal and visceral surfaces to become rough. This produces a rubbing or grating sound heard with the stethoscope. Pericardial friction rub is often heard loudest of the apex and usual covers systole and diastole (Seidel *et al.*, 2003)
  - *prosthetic valves* produce loud clicks during opening and closure.

- Murmurs - palpation of the precordium may have provided some clues about the heart that can be considered during auscultation. A forceful left ventricular beat may be because of aortic or mitral valve disease so listening carefully for a murmur is important. Murmurs are generally caused by some disruption in blood flow into, through or out of the heart. Diseased valves that either do not open or close normally are the most common causes of murmurs. Other reasons for murmurs may include high output states (thyrotoxicosis, pregnancy), structural defects, altered blood flow in major vessels near the heart, obstructive disease in cervical arteries and vigorous left ventricular ejection (Seidel et al., 2003). A full examination as well as other diagnostic testing is useful in accurate diagnosis of a murmur. Murmurs are classified according to timing (systole or diastole), pitch, intensity, pattern, quality, location, radiation and relationship to respiration (Tables 3.1 and 3.2).

Peripheral arteries and veins

Palpation of radial and carotid pulses, measurement of blood pressure, and examination of JVP has been discussed above. A full examination of the vascular system should be completed, even if there were no obvious initial signs, to gain a clear picture of the state of the cardiovascular system (Munro and Campbell, 2003). This part of the examination should be performed in a systematic way that is comfortable for the examiner.

- Peripheral pulses - palpate pulses and compare with opposite side:
  - brachial - medial to biceps tendon
  - radial - medial and ventral side of the wrist

Table 3.1 Gradation of murmurs

Grade 1	Very faint, may be barely audible with a stethoscope in a quiet room
Grade 2	Quiet, but heard when the stethoscope is placed over the heart
Grade 3	Moderately loud
Grade 4	Loud, with palpable thrill
Grade 5	Very loud, thrill palpated easily
Grade 6	Audible when stethoscope not in contact with chest wall, thrill palpated easily

Adapted from Bickley (2004). Reproduced with permission from John Wiley & Sons Ltd.

Table 3.2 Timing of murmurs

Timing	Likely causes
Midsystolic ▯▲▯ S_1 S_2	Innocent murmurs (no cardiovascular abnormality) Physiologic murmur (pregnancy, sepsis, anaemia) Aortic stenosis or aortic sclerosis Pulmonic stenosis Hypertrophic cardiomyopathy
Pansystolic ▯—▯ S_1 S_2	Mitral regurgitation Tricuspid regurgitation Ventricular septal defect
Late systolic ▯◢▯ S_1 S_2	Mitral valve prolapse Hypertrophic cardiomyopathy Coarctation of aorta
Early diastolic ▯ ▯◣▯ S_1 S_2 S_1	Aortic regurgitation Pulmonary regurgitation
Mid-late diastolic ▯ ▯___▯ S_1 S_2 S_1	Mitral stenosis Tricuspid stenosis

Adapted from Kumar and Clark (2005). Reproduced with permission from John Wiley & Sons Ltd.

- femoral – may be difficult to palpate in obese patients but helpful to identify any potential problems if this route is to be used for access in coronary angiography
- popliteal – popliteal fossa – helpful if the patient is prone with knee flexed

- dorsalis pedis - medial side of the dorsum of the foot with foot slightly dorsiflexed
- posterior tibial - behind and just inferior to medial malleolus of the ankle
- abdominal aorta - press on both sides of the aorta, feeling for any lateral pulsation suggestive of an aneurysm.
- Auscultation - bruits are caused by turbulent blood flow due to constriction or altered flow. Use a stethoscope to listen over major blood vessels for the presence of a bruit. Sites to auscultate include:
  - abdominal aorta - if there are clinical signs of aortic aneurysm
  - femoral arteries - if there are signs of peripheral arterial disease in lower limb.

Chest pain assessment

Chest pain is a common reason for people to seek healthcare advice within the primary and secondary care setting (Cayley, 2005). It is a symptom most commonly associated with heart disease, but may also be present in many different disease processes (Kumar and Clark, 2005). Chest pain may be present in acute coronary syndromes (ACS), but patients with pulmonary or gastrointestinal problems may also present with chest pain, as well as those with trauma or soft tissue injury (Table 3.3). A thorough history and clinical examination will help the practitioner make a correct diagnosis.

History taking

The history will help to clearly establish the character of the symptoms in order to distinguish between chest pain from myocardial ischaemia and non-ischaemic or non-cardiac chest pain. There are five factors that may help in determining which patients are having pain related to an acute coronary syndrome: the nature of the pain, a prior history of heart disease, gender, age and the number of traditional risk factors present (Braunwald et al., 2002). Initial questions should be broad, such as "Do you have pain or discomfort in your chest?" Further questions should elicit the attributes of the pain (Bickley and Szilagyi. 2009).

- Onset - "When did you first notice the pain?"
- Provocation - "What kinds of activities bring on the pain?" "Do you have other symptoms such as shortness of breath, sweating, nausea or fast heart beat?"
- Quality - "What is it like?" Ask patients to use their own words to describe the pain.
- Radiation - "Where is it?" "Does it radiate?" Chest pain symptoms are varied and may be poorly localised. Ask the patient to point to the area of discomfort.

Table 3.3 Chest pain

Differential diagnosis of chest pain	Common signs presentation
Acute coronary syndromes	• Varied presentation across anterior chest and may be radiating to neck, jaw, shoulders or arms • Described as "pressing, squeezing, tightness, heaviness or burning" • May occur with exertion or at rest depending on degree of myocardial ischaemia • May be relieved by rest or require nitroglycerine or morphine • Sometimes accompanied by dyspnoea, sweating, nausea
Aortic aneurysm/ dissection	• Anterior chest pain radiating to back, abdomen or neck • Severe with a "ripping" or "tearing" feeling • Usual starts abruptly and persistent • May also have syncope, hemiplegia or paraplegia
Pericarditis/ myocarditis	• Usually in the precordial area with radiation to the shoulder tip and neck • Described as "sharp" or "knifelike" • Tends to be persistent and aggravated by breathing, coughing, lying down and changing position • Position changes may give some relief
Pleurisy	• Discomfort in chest wall overlying area of inflammation • Often severe, persistent • Described as "sharp, knifelike" • Aggravated by coughing, movements of the thorax • Lying on the involved side may provide some relief • May also be associated with other symptoms of pneumonia, pulmonary infarction or neoplasm
Oesophagogastric disorders	• Typically just behind the sternum, may radiate to back • Described as "burning, squeezing" and symptoms may be similar to angina • Tends to be unpredictable and variable onset • Aggravated by large meals, lying down or bending over. Activity does not tend to exacerbate the discomfort • May be relieved by antacids
Chest wall pain (costochondritis)	• May be related to a minor injury and can be anywhere along costal cartilages or elsewhere in the thorax • Severity is variable and feels like a stabbing, sticking, aching discomfort • May be aggravated by movement of the chest, arms and trunk • There may be localised tenderness

Adapted from Bickley and Szilagyi (2008).

- Relief – "What do you do to make it better?"
- Severity – "How bad is it?" A pain scale may be helpful.
- Timing – "When does (did) it start?" "How long does it last?" "How often does it occur?" Patients having an ACS may have severe discomfort that comes on quickly or gradually and usually lasts for more than 20 minutes (Wallentin *et al.*, 2002).

Risk factors should be established for all patients presenting with chest pain. This will help in making a diagnosis. Major risk factors for cardiac disease include personal history of ischaemic heart disease, family history of ischaemic heart disease, smoking, diabetes, hypertension and hypercholesterolaemia. The more major risk factors that are present, the more likely the disease becomes (this is discussed further in Chapter 4).

Clinical examination

The immediate examination of any patient presenting with chest pain is focused on determining if symptoms are life-threatening (Erhardt *et al.*, 2002). Myocardial ischaemia and infarction may quickly lead to cardiac arrest. Recognising and responding to early signs and symptoms of cardiac problems may prevent a cardiac arrest (ILCOR, 2005). The following approach in parallel with the history and cardiac examination may be used to quickly assess the patient (Smith *et al.*, 2002).

- Airway – assess for any signs of airway obstruction and treat airway obstruction as an emergency. Administer oxygen at a high concentration as soon as possible.
- Breathing – look, listen and feel for signs of breathing problems. An increased breathing rate may be the first physiological observation to alter in the deteriorating patient (Smith *et al.*, 2002). Count the respiratory rate while assessing the depth and pattern of breathing. Life-threatening conditions (acute severe asthma, pneumothorax and pulmonary oedema) must be treated immediately. Provide breaths with a pocket mask or bag-mask to any patient who has stopped breathing or has inadequate breathing.
- Circulation – do a rapid general examination of the patient noting colour of hands and feet and temperature of the hands. Measure CRT. Take a blood pressure and look for other signs of decreased cardiac output such as a change in level of consciousness. Any patient with a suspected ACS should be treated initially with oxygen, aspirin, nitroglycerine and morphine. A 12-lead ECG should be recorded.
- Disability – assess the patient's conscious level quickly using AVPU: **A**lert, responds to **V**ocal stimuli, responds to **P**ainful stimuli or **U**nresponsive. Hypoxia, hypercapnia and cerebral hypoperfusion are common causes of unconsciousness.

- Exposure – look at the patient exposed from head to toe and consider anything else that may be causing chest pain (e.g. injury, trauma).

Once the patient is stabilised a full cardiovascular examination as described above can be completed. In some cases, the initial exam will be unremarkable and a diagnosis is made based on the reported history. In many cases, further testing will be required. The following sections will discuss electrocardiography, laboratory testing and diagnostic procedures.

Electrocardiography

The 12-lead ECG is used frequently in primary and secondary care settings. It is a cheap, non-invasive and rapid investigation that is widely used for patients presenting with chest pain. Acute coronary syndromes, pulmonary embolism, pericarditis and aortic dissection may cause ECG changes. However, the ECG may also be normal in these conditions so the reading must be interpreted along with the history and clinical examination (ECG recording and interpretation is discussed in detail in Chapter 10).

The 12-lead ECG should be recorded as soon as possible during the initial assessment of the patient with chest pain. It is a crucial part of risk assessment and planning of treatment. The main focus of 12-lead ECG interpretation during the initial assessment is to diagnose the underlying rhythm using the approach described above and determine if there are changes related to myocardial ischaemia. Where in the myocardium the ischaemia is happening will determine which leads on the 12-lead ECG show changes.

- Acute ST segment elevation in a patient with a history and clinical findings of an acute myocardial infarction is an indication for immediate treatment to try to re-open an occluded coronary artery (coronary reperfusion). This will be with percutaneous coronary intervention or thrombolytic therapy. The diagnosis is ST elevation myocardial infarction (STEMI).
- ST segment depression indicates that ischaemia is occurring, but the patient is not likely to benefit from immediate reperfusion therapy. The diagnosis is either unstable angina or non-ST elevation myocardial infarction (NSTEMI). Higher-risk patients may need immediate medical treatment (e.g. low molecular weight heparin, aspirin, clopidogrel, beta blockade, glycoprotein IIb/IIIa inhibitor), prompt investigation with coronary angiography and in some cases PCI or coronary bypass surgery.

Laboratory tests

There is a range of blood tests commonly done in primary and secondary care settings to evaluate patients with chest pain. Common tests include a full blood count (FBC), urea and electrolytes (U&Es), lipid profiles and cardiac markers. The results of most testing will not alter the immediate clinical management with the exception of cardiac markers.

Cardiac markers

Serum cardiac troponin (I and T) is a very useful tool for determining the presence and extent of myocardial ischaemia. The clinical history, 12-lead ECG and cardiac troponin results are considered to be the key markers in diagnosing an acute coronary syndrome (Bertrand et al., 2002).

- Cardiac troponin is found in myocardial cells and can be detected in the serum within 4 hours of ischaemic injury. They may remain elevated for up to one week, but troponin levels are most reliable 8–12 hours after onset of the patient's worst pain (James et al., 2005).
- Elevated troponin is also useful in predicting adverse outcomes. The higher the level of troponin, the greater the risk of death and re-infarction (Antman et al., 2004).
- Normal troponin levels are determined by local laboratories.
- Troponin may be elevated in significant pulmonary embolism, cardiac contusion, heart failure or renal failure (Thygesen et al., 2007). The results should always be interpreted in light of clinical history and examination findings.
- Other cardiac biochemical markers may be used and include creatine kinase (CK), CK-MB (an isoenzyme of CK) and myoglobin.

Diagnostic procedures

Chest X-ray

Chest radiography is often done if the patient presents to the hospital with chest pain. Patients with ACS generally have a normal chest X-ray. Abnormal radiographic findings such as pulmonary oedema or increased cardiac ratio from left ventricular dilatation may provide further diagnostic information for patients presenting with cardiac symptoms. A chest X-ray is also important for patients presenting with traumatic chest pain to identify a fracture, haemothorax, pneumothorax, pericardial effusion, mediastinal injury or diaphragmatic rupture.

Echocardiography

An echocardiogram (ECHO) is useful for identifying abnormalities in the myocardial wall that occur from ischaemia and necrosis. There is limited usefulness for an ECHO in the acute phase of an acute coronary syndrome.

However, the ECHO may be valuable in detecting an aortic dissection or pulmonary embolus.

Exercise tolerance testing

The exercise tolerance test is generally used for patients who present with chest pain but do not have:

- pain during the period of observation
- ST segment depression or ST segment elevation
- elevated troponin (or other cardiac biochemical markers).

These patients are considered to be at low risk for developing adverse events such as myocardial infarction or death (Bertrand *et al.*, 2002). The exercise test is useful for determining whether the underlying cause of chest pain is related to cardiac disease. The Bruce protocol is the most widely adopted protocol and consists of seven stages of three minutes each (Hill and Timmis, 2003). The modified Bruce protocol may be used for patients following a myocardial infarction or who have difficulty with mobility. A highly abnormal exercise test result is an indication for urgent further investigation (SIGN, 2007).

Myocardial perfusion scintigraphy (MPS)

Myocardial perfusion scintigraphy with exercise or pharmacologic stress is another non-invasive investigation that can detect the presence of coronary heart disease (SIGN, 2007). It is particularly useful for patients who have pre-existing ECG abnormalities, unusual patterns in the electrical activity in the heart or those who are not able to exercise.

Coronary angiography

Coronary angiography is an invasive procedure to view the coronary arteries and determine the nature, anatomy and severity of coronary artery disease. As well as providing diagnostic imaging of the coronary arteries, the valvular and left ventricular function can also be determined. SIGN (2007) recommends that angiography should be considered in patients who are at high risk or where a diagnosis remains unclear after non-invasive testing.

Summary

Clinical examination skills are essential when considering patients with cardiac problems, the emphasis is upon using a systematic approach to ensure a thorough and timely examination and assessment. General techniques of inspection, palpation, percussion and auscultation need skill and understanding to perfect and perform with confidence, but are essential to the nurse working within cardiac care.

References

Antman EM, Anbe DT, Armstrong PW et al. (2004) ACC/AHA guidelines for the management of patients with ST-elevation myocardial infarction: a report of the American College or Cardiology/American Heart Association Task Force on Practice Guidelines. Writing Committee to revise the 1999 guidelines for the management of patients with acute myocardial infarction. *Journal of the American College of Cardiology* **44**(3): 671–719.

Bertrand ME, Simoons ML and Fox KAA (2002) Management of acute coronary syndromes in patients presenting without persistent ST-segment elevation. *European Heart Journal* **23**: 1809–40.

Bickley L and Szilagyi P (2008) *Bates' Guide to Physical Examination and History Taking*. Philadelphia, Lippincott Williams and Wilkins.

Braunwald E, Antman EM, Beasley JW, Califf RM and Cheitlin MD (2002) ACC/AHA 2002 guideline update for the management of patients with unstable angina and non-ST-segment elevation myocardial infarction. *Journal of the American College of Cardiology* **40**: 1366–74.

Cayley WE (2005) Diagnosing the cause of chest pain. *American Family Physician* **72**(10): 2012–21.

Cox C (2004) *Physical Assessment for Nurses*. Oxford, Blackwell.

Erhardt L, Herlitz J, Bossart L et al. (2002) Task Force report on the management of chest pain. *European Heart Journal* **23**(15): 1153–76.

Guyton AC and Hall JE (2000) *Textbook of Medical Physiology*. Philadelphia, W B Saunders.

Hill J and Timmis A (2003) Exercise tolerance testing. In: Morris F, Edhouse J, Brady WJ and Camm J (eds) *ABC of Clinical Electrocardiography*, pp. 41–5. London, BMJ Publishing Group.

International Liaison Committee on Resuscitation (2005) International consensus on cardiopulmonary resuscitation and ememrgency cardiovascular science with treatment recommendations. *Resuscitation* **67**: 187–211.

James SK, Lindahl B and Wallentin LC (2005) Biomarkers for risk stratification in non-ST segment elevation acute coronary syndromes: what is their relation to classical clinical characteristics? In: Ferrari R and Hearse DJ (eds) *Dialogues in Cardiovascular Medicine – Acute Coronary Syndromes* **10**(3): 153–62.

Kumar P and Clark M (2005) *Clinical Medicine*. Oxford, Elsevier Saunders.

Longmore M, Wilkinson I, Turmezei T and Cheung C (2007) *Oxford Handbook of Clinical Medicine*. Oxford, Oxford University Press.

Moule P and Albarran J (2009) *Practical Resuscitation for Healthcare Professionals*. Oxford, Wiley-Blackwell.

Munro J and Campbell I (2003) *Macleod's Clinical Examination*. London, Churchill Livingstone.

Scottish Intercollegiate Guideline Network (SIGN) (2007) *Cardiac Rehabilitation. A quick reference guide*. www.sign.ac.uk (accessed September 2009).

Seidel H, Ball J, Dains J and Benedict GW (2003) *Mosby's Guide to Clinical Examination*. St Louis, Mosby.

Smith G, Osgood V and Crane S (2002) ALERT – a multiprofessional training course in the care of the acutely ill adult patient. *Resuscitation* **52**: 281-6.

Thygesen K, Alpert JS and White HD (2007) Universal definition of myocardial infarction. *European Heart Journal* **28**(20): 2525-38.

Wallentin L, Bertil L and Siegbahn A (2002) Unstable coronary artery disease Section 2. In: Crawford MH and DiMarco JP (eds) *Cardiology*, pp. 13.1-13.19. London, Mosby.

Chapter 4

Diagnosing Acute Coronary Syndrome

John McGowan

Introduction

The initial diagnosis of an acute coronary syndrome (ACS) is based entirely on history, risk factors and, to a lesser extent, changes in the electrocardiograph (ECG). Patients with an ACS include those with a clinical presentation of one of the following range of diagnoses: unstable angina, non-ST segment elevation myocardial infarction (NSTEMI) and ST segment elevation myocardial infarction (STEMI). This spectrum of ACS is a useful framework for developing therapeutic strategies. The aim of this chapter is to understand the assessment process of a patient presenting with ACS and the investigations that aid its diagnosis and subsequent categorisation.

Learning outcomes

At the end of this chapter the reader will be able to:

- describe the significance of undertaking a patient history to establish a diagnosis of ACS
- describe the assessment of a patient using an ABCDE approach
- discuss the significance of 12-lead ECG interpretation to establish the diagnosis of ACS
- describe the common biochemical markers used in the diagnosis of ACS
- discuss the clinical significance of risk stratification.

Nursing the Cardiac Patient, First Edition. Edited by Melanie Humphreys.
© 2011 Blackwell Publishing Ltd. Published 2011 by Blackwell Publishing Ltd.

Acute coronary syndromes in perspective

The type of ACS is confirmed on the basis of the following diagnostic criteria:

- clinical presentation and history of an acute cardiac event
- changes in the morphology of the ECG which suggest an acute cardiac event
- elevated levels of biochemical markers in their blood.

In general, if the patient has two of these three diagnostic features, they can be diagnosed as having had an acute coronary syndrome. A history of strong risk factors for coronary heart disease (CHD) may confirm the likelihood of an acute cardiac event.

The rapid assessment and diagnosis of an ACS allows early revascularisation, either by percutaneous coronary intervention (PCI), thrombolysis or coronary artery bypass grafting (CABG), to be carried out. In STEMI these procedures must be carried out within a few hours to have any benefit (see Chapter 7). It is currently recommended that patients whose symptoms suggest it is less than 12 hours since the onset of an acute MI should be considered for these treatments (SIGN 93); NSTEMI may be treated some days after the event. There is consistent evidence that the longer the delay to revascularisation, the greater the number of deaths (van de Werf et al., 2003). For this reason, treatment is initiated on the basis of presentation and the presence or absence of ECG changes and is not delayed by waiting for biochemical markers, which may not be elevated for up to 12 hours (discussed further below).

Presentation

Typically, the patient presenting with an ACS will show some or all of the following signs and symptoms (see Chapter 3 for further details):

- chest pain often accompanied by pain or numbness in the left arm or jaw
- nausea and vomiting
- diaphoresis (grey and clammy)
- breathlessness
- collapse
- arrhythmias or cardiac arrest.

Chest pain

Chest pain is the most common symptom of the patient experiencing ACS. It is caused by ischaemia, where the oxygen demand in the myocardium exceeds the oxygen supplied by the coronary circulation. Patients with an ACS will often describe the pain using the following expressions: tight, crushing, like a band or belt round the chest, heavy, like a weight on the chest.

These are descriptions of what is commonly referred to as cardiac chest pain. This pain will typically last more than 20 minutes (Thygesen et al., 2007). Pain that gets worse when the patient breathes in (pleuritic type pain) is much less likely to be caused by an acute coronary syndrome.

Pain in the chest may be accompanied by pain and numbness in other areas, typically the left arm and jaw. Occasionally pain will go to the patient's back, right arm or legs, or may be epigastric.

The intensity of the pain can vary. For some patients it is the worst pain they have ever felt, for others it may be merely uncomfortable. Some patients may not experience pain at all. Women, non-smokers, diabetic and older patients may have little or no pain as a presenting symptom (Culic, 2002).

Nausea and vomiting

Patients are commonly nauseated and will often vomit. This is due to a combination of increased autonomic activity (see below) and the systemic effects of stimulation of receptors in the left ventricular wall, the Bezold-Jarisch reflex (Sleight, 1981).

Diaphoresis

Increased circulating levels of the catecholamines adrenaline and noradrenaline, mobilised by pain, fear, diminished cardiac output or in response to injured myocardium cause arteriolar vasoconstriction. The reduction in blood flow to the skin causes it to appear pale or grey, and the patient's peripheries will be cool to touch. Increased sweating induced by noradrenaline makes the skin to feel clammy.

Breathlessness

Damage to the left ventricle may reduce its efficiency as a pump and reduce the flow of blood from the pulmonary circulation. Engorgement of the pulmonary veins makes the lungs less compliant which will make the patient feel that they are working harder to breath.

Collapse

For many years it has been recognised that autonomic disturbance frequently occurs at the onset of an ACS. Increased parasympathetic activity causing profound bradycardias, and increased sympathetic activity causing tachyarrhythmias, may occur, either of which can cause collapse (Webb et al., 1972). Reduced cardiac output due to left ventricular impairment may also cause collapse.

Arrhythmias or cardiac arrest

Sudden cardiac arrest or cardiac death is a common presentation and acute coronary syndromes are the most common cause of malignant ventricular arrhythmias (Arntz et al., 2005). This is further discussed in Chapter 10.

Assessment

As the risk of arrhythmias and cardiac arrest is highest in the first few hours, assessment of patients with suspected ACS should be carried out in an area with rapid access to a defibrillator and other resuscitation equipment, and by staff skilled in their use.

Assessment of the patient with a suspected acute coronary event will comprise:

- a rapid assessment of ABCDE, including recording vital signs (detailed assessment of the cardiovascular system is covered in more detail in Chapter 3)
- taking a focused history
- investigations.

ABCDE evaluation

Airway: if the patient can talk, their upper airway is clear. If their conscious level is impaired, there is upper airway noise or they are unable to verbalise, then simple airway opening techniques should be used. Oxygen should be administered according to local protocols.

Breathing: the respiratory rate should be recorded. Tachypnoea and bradypnoea are powerful markers of serious illness. Their work of breathing should be noted, including use of accessory muscles and signs of respiratory distress. Depth of respiration should be noted and whether both sides of their chest are moving. Pulse oximetry should be monitored.

Circulation: the radial pulse should be palpated and rate recorded, and the patient's peripheral perfusion and colour noted. Cardiac monitoring should be started, the blood pressure should be recorded, an intravenous cannula inserted and bloods taken.

Disability: the patient's conscious level should be assessed, using the AVPU scale. Are they **A**lert, do they respond to **V**oice, respond to **P**ain or are they **U**nresponsive. If they don't respond to voice or better, their pupil size and reaction to light should be noted. A bedside blood glucose test should be performed.

Exposure: the patient should be undressed and systematically examined for any injuries, rashes, oedema or other skin signs. Their temperature should be taken.

Patient history

The history taken from the patient should be rapid and focused. It should allow the nurse to assess the likelihood of the patient having an ACS and their risk of deterioration. Questions will include:

- the nature of any chest pain and when it started
- any other symptoms associated with it

- any previous episodes of chest pain
- any previous illnesses, especially diabetes
- any allergies
- what drugs the patient is taking, prescribed and non-prescribed, including smoking history
- family history of heart disease.

Investigations

A 12-lead ECG should be performed as soon as possible. Venous blood should be sent off for urea and electrolytes, liver function tests, troponin (see below), full blood count, glucose and an inflammatory marker such as C-reactive protein. If the patient has signs of respiratory distress or desaturation on oximetry, an arterial blood gas sample may be taken. A portable chest X-ray should be requested. If the patient has had any back pain, their radial pulses should be compared and their blood pressure checked in both arms. A large difference between the right and left sides would suggest they might have a thoracic aortic aneurysm.

Interpreting the 12-lead ECG

The 12-lead ECG is a simple non-invasive bedside test that can confirm the diagnosis of an ACS and allow this to be categorised as an STEMI, a NSTEMI or as unstable angina. It can be readily repeated to give a dynamic picture of the response to reperfusion strategies, and the initial ECG provides a baseline against which serial ECGs can be compared.

The ECG is a surface plot of changes in voltage in the heart (vertical axis) against time (horizontal axis). Each component of the ECG complex, the P wave, QRS complex and T waves can be related to electrical activity within the conduction system of the heart (Figure 4.1).

The rules that determine which wave is which are as follows, remembering that not all of these waves may be seen in all leads or indeed, be present.

- The small, generally positive (i.e. above the baseline) wave just before the main complex is the P wave.
- If the first deflection of the main complex is negative (i.e. below the baseline) this is the Q wave.
- If the first deflection of the main complex is positive, then it is the R wave. Otherwise the R wave is the first positive deflection after the Q wave.
- The S wave is a downward deflection following the R wave. This may not always go below the baseline.
- The final, normally positive, deflection in the complex is the T wave.

Relating these waves to activity within the heart, the P wave is produced by atrial depolarisation, the QRS by ventricular depolarisation and the T wave by repolarisation in the ventricles.

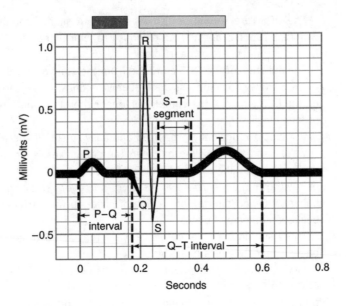

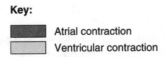

Key:

■ Atrial contraction
☐ Ventricular contraction

Figure 4.1 The ECG complex with the PQRS and T waves labelled. From Tortora GJ and Derrickson BH (2009) *Principles of Anatomy and Physiology* (12e). Reproduced with permission from John Wiley & Sons.

When reading a 12-lead ECG a systematic approach makes it easier to describe any changes and reduces the likelihood of changes being missed. First, decide what the heart rhythm is by answering five questions.

• What is the QRS rate?
• Is the QRS rhythm regular or irregular?
• Is the QRS width normal or broad?
• Is atrial activity present? If so, are these P waves? Is there other atrial activity?
• How is atrial activity related to ventricular activity?

The QRS rate can be determined by counting how many large squares on the ECG paper there are between each QRS complex and dividing this into 300, or by taking the patient's pulse. It is unwise to rely on a machine estimate of the heart rate, e.g. from an oximeter or an ECG monitor. The normal heart rate should be between 50 and 100 beats per minute. Generally, tachycardias above 150 are abnormal tachycardias. Bradycardias below 40 are generally abnormal, although people who exercise regularly may have slow resting heart rates.

The QRS rate should be grossly regular. A slight irregularity associated with respiration is normal, but obvious irregularity may be due to atrial fibrillation, ectopic beats or heart block.

The duration of the QRS complex, from the start of the Q wave to the end of the S wave should be less than 120 milliseconds. This is three small squares on the ECG paper. If the complex is longer than this, there may be a bundle branch block.

P waves are normally organised and easy to see. If there are no obvious P waves and the baseline between the complexes is irregular or flat, the rhythm is most likely to be atrial fibrillation. P waves, either normal-looking or sawtooth in appearance at a rate of one every small square on the ECG paper (300 per minute), are a sign of atrial flutter. Atrial activity is usually best seen in leads II or V_1.

There should normally be one P wave for each QRS complex. More than one is suggestive of a heart block.

Having established the heart rhythm, the next step in interpreting a 12-lead ECG is to look at each lead in turn. Each of the 12 leads of the ECG can be thought of as providing an electrical "view" of the heart. The views provided by these leads are:

- leads II, III and aVF look at the inferior surface of the heart
- lead I looks at the antero-apical surface of the heart
- lead aVL looks at the left lateral side of the heart
- lead V_1 looks at the atria, leads $V_{2,3,4}$ at the intraventricular septum, leads $V_{5,6}$ at the lateral surface of the heart
- lead aVR is an unusual lead, but ST segment elevation in this is a marker of widespread myocardial ischaemia (Williamson et al., 2006).

When looking at each lead in turn:

- look at the ST segments, are these elevated or depressed? T waves, are these upright, flat or inverted? Look for pathological Q waves. When inspecting the T waves it is useful to note that they should be the same way around as the QRS complex, i.e. it is normal for the T wave to be inverted in lead aVr as the QRS is negative and at times in leads III and V_1
- if the QRS duration is prolonged, decide whether there is a right bundle branch block (large R wave in V_1 or V_2) or left bundle branch block (large R wave in V_5 or V_6)
- look at the chest leads for normal R wave progression
- estimate the electrical axis. Look at leads I and II: these should be positive. If lead I is mainly negative there is right axis deviation, if lead II is mainly negative, left axis deviation.

In general, significant ST segment elevation indicates acute myocardial injury, such as a myocardial infarction (STEMI). Significant ST segment elevation is defined as being 1mm or more above the baseline in the limb leads

(leads I, II, III, aVR, aVL, aVF) or 2 mm or more in the chest leads (leads V_1 to V_6). ST segment elevation myocardial infarction is shown by significant ST elevation in two or more contiguous leads. That is, in leads looking at the same part of the heart: leads II, II or aVF, leads I or aVL or adjacent leads in leads V_1 to V_6 (Thygesen et al., 2007).

ST segment depression is a sign of ischaemia. T waves that are flattened or inverted may indicate recent myocardial damage, although some drugs, such as digoxin, can cause changes in the T waves. Deeply inverted T waves may indicate a partial thickness or sub-endocardial myocardial infarction (NSTEMI).

Pathological Q waves may be defined to be longer than 30 milliseconds (1/2 small squares of the ECG paper) or deeper than 2 mm (two small squares of the ECG paper). In health, there is often a deep Q wave in lead III, but this can disappear on deep inspiration. Pathological Q waves indicate myocardial necrosis, either recent or healed.

New left or right bundle branch block may indicate myocardial damage. Left bundle branch block makes diagnosing myocardial infarction from the ECG difficult.

Normally in the chest leads, there is no R wave in V_1 but it will be present in V_3 and get bigger in each lead round to V_6. If there is no R wave in V_3 and V_4, it is equivalent to having Q waves in the chest leads, indicating recent or healed myocardial necrosis.

The cardiac axis may be shifted to the right or left by a variety of conditions including pulmonary embolus, cardiomyopathy and bundle branch block.

ECGs in acute coronary syndromes

See Figures 4.2 to 4.5.

Biochemical markers

When subjected to ischaemia, cardiac myocytes initially shut down, then die (necrosis). When cell death occurs, the cell membrane disintegrates and the cell contents are released. These cell contents are the basis of biochemical markers. This process does not happen instantly; it may be up to 4 hours before cell death occurs (ESC) and longer before the contents reach the bloodstream.

It should be noted that rises in biochemical markers alone merely indicate cell death and not the mechanism. These will rise in response to, among other causes, direct trauma, heart failure and pulmonary embolism.

In health, low levels of these biochemical markers are present in the blood, reflecting apoptosis and other factors causing cell death, which are a normal part of life. Each laboratory will have established levels, known as

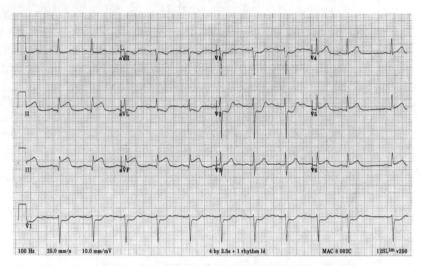

Figure 4.2 Infero-lateral ST segment elevation myocardial infarction. The rhythm is sinus with a short sino-atrial pause just before the last complex on the ECG. There is ST segment elevation in leads II, III, aVF, V₅ and V₆. There is ST depression in leads I, aVL, V₁ and V₂. There is a pathological Q wave in lead III.

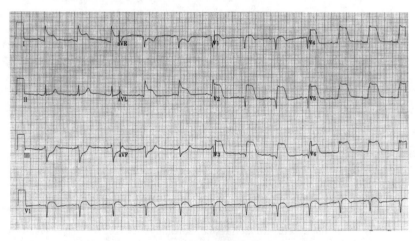

Figure 4.3 Extensive antero-lateral ST segment elevation myocardial infarction. The rhythm is sinus. There is ST segment elevation in leads I, aVL, V₂ to V₆. There is ST segment depression in leads III, aVR and aVF. There is no R wave in V₃.

the normal reference range, that occur in health. This range may vary from lab to lab, depending on which testing kits are used.

For many years, elevated levels of transaminase enzymes in the patient's blood were used in the diagnosis of MI. These enzyme levels were slow to rise, meaning patients often had repeated blood sampling, and were not specific to cardiac tissue. More recently the transfer enzyme creatine phos-

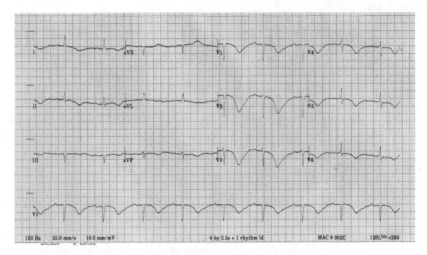

Figure 4.4 Non-ST segment elevation MI, an anterior sub-endocardial myocardial infarction. The rhythm is sinus bradycardia with T wave inversion in leads I, II, III, aVR, aVF and V_1 to V_6. The deep T inversion in V_2 and V_3 is suggestive of infarction.

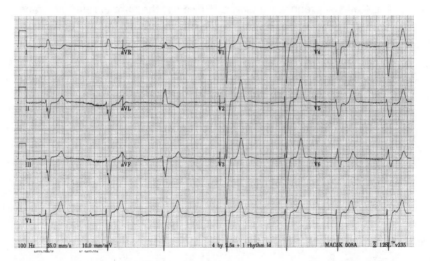

Figure 4.5 Left bundle branch block. The rhythm is complete heart block, the QRS duration is 160 milliseconds (four small squares). The largest R wave in the chest leads is in V_6.

phokinase (CK-MB) was used. However, this has largely been superseded by the cardiac specific troponins.

Creatine phosphokinase

This enzyme is found widely in body tissues. There are five isoenzymes of creatine phosphokinase, all varying in their sub-unit structure. The type

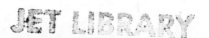

present at greater concentrations in myocytes is the MB variant (short for muscle-brain). This is usually abbreviated to CK-MB. The levels of this enzyme rise within a few hours and return to normal levels by 72 hours. Elevated levels of CK-MB may also be found in conditions such as heart failure, stroke and where there is extensive muscle damage. Use of this assay in the diagnosis of ACS is now confined to those facilities where troponin levels cannot be assayed. Blood samples should be obtained for CK-MB on admission and at 6 to 12 hours after the onset of acute symptoms. A level greater than 400 U/l is indicative of myocardial necrosis (Fox *et al.*, 2004).

Troponin

Troponins are regulatory proteins closely involved in the contractile apparatus of muscle cells. There are a number of isoforms of this protein, of which troponin I and troponin T are those found in cardiac muscle. In addition to being sensitive markers for myocyte necrosis, the extent of the rise in troponin levels has been shown to have a predictive value of adverse clinical events and is used as part of risk stratification of patients following an ACS. Both troponin I and troponin T perform similarly as markers of tissue damage and as prognostic markers. However, the normal reference ranges of these proteins are different. Troponin levels sampled at 12 hours after the acute cardiac event are highly sensitive and specific of myocardial damage (Ebell *et al.*, 2000). However, around half of patients with an ACS will have elevated troponin levels on admission. For this reason, blood samples should be obtained on admission and at 12 hours after the precipitating event. Those patients with elevated troponins at admission can have earlier confirmation of the diagnosis and risk stratification.

The extent of the rise in troponins equates well with the extent of tissue damage. No rise would suggest no myocyte death, a small rise indicates that there are small areas of myocardial necrosis and larger rises indicate myocardial infarction. While examples of different levels for these clinical events have been published (Fox *et al.*, 2004), there will be differences between laboratories, so reference needs to be made to the specific guidelines and thresholds from the lab that processes the sample.

Tying together the diagnosis

When information about the patient's presentation, ECG changes and troponin levels is available, their acute coronary syndrome can be categorised. This is summarised in Figure 4.6. These categories assume a history of an acute cardiac event.

Risk stratification

It is clear from Figure 4.6 that a combination of ECG changes and troponin levels can give an estimate of the patient's risk of death. However, they may

Disease category	ECG changes	Troponin level	
ACS with unstable angina	ST depression, T inversion or transient ST elevation	Normal	Increasing amount of myocardial damage*
ACS with myocyte necrosis	ST depression, T inversion or transient ST elevation	Slightly elevated	Increasing risk of death within 6 months
ACS with clinical myocardial infarction	ST elevation or depression, or T inversion; Q waves may evolve	Significantly elevated	

Figure 4.6 Categorising acute coronary syndromes (adapted from Fox *et al.*, 2004). It is worth noting that ST depression causes the longest-term risk rather than ST elevation. When STEMI is treated its risk becomes low; ST depression, however, can mean widespread coronary disease, which can have a long-term mortality risk.

have other factors that will worsen their prognosis. For example, a patient with a new clinical MI who has had four previous infarctions is likely to have a worse prognosis than someone who is having their first. There have been a number of tools proposed that use multiple indices to stratify the patient's risk of death or other adverse events. There are two main reasons for risk stratification. First, it identifies which patients are at high risk in order that early interventions can be applied to reduce that risk. Patients with a greater than 10% risk of death or infarction at one year benefit from invasive revascularisation. Those with a risk less than this do not seem to benefit (Fox *et al.*, 2005). Second, it allows valid comparisons to be made in research studies. There have been a large number of studies carried out on interventions, for example thrombolysis and angioplasty in ACS. One criticism of many of these studies is that mortality rates in the study groups are lower than those seen in clinical practice. By declaring the relative risk in these studies, selection bias can be assessed.

There are a number of risk stratification tools available, of which that produced from the GRACE registry is best for accuracy and reproducibility (Granger *et al.*, 2003). Scores are assigned to eight parameters:

- grade of heart failure
- systolic BP
- heart rate
- age
- creatinine
- cardiac arrest

> ## Box 4.1 TIMI (thrombolysis in myocardial infarction) risk score for unstable angina/non-ST-segment elevation myocardial infarction
>
> If present, each of the following contributes +1 to the overall score.
>
> - Score >4 indicates high-risk non-ST-segment elevation ACS.
> - Age ≥65 years.
> - At least three risk factors for coronary artery disease: male sex, hyperlipidaemia, hypertension, smoking, diabetes mellitus, family history of premature coronary disease.
> - Previous coronary stenosis ≥50 per cent.
> - ST-segment elevation or depression at presentation.
> - Two or more anginal events in the past 24 hours.
> - Aspirin use in the past 7 days.
> - Elevated serum cardiac biomarkers.
>
> (Antman et al., 2000)

- ST segment elevation
- cardiac enzymes.

The sum of these scores is matched with a likelihood of in-hospital death. An online tool is available to calculate this risk (see Web resources).

It is risk status that drives pharmacological treatments and the timing of further interventional procedures; the TIMI score is also a commonly used risk stratification tool (Antman et al., 2000; see Box 4.1).

Imaging techniques

Coronary angiography

Coronary angiography gives direct visual evidence of the presence and extent of impairment to blood flow in the coronary arteries. It has the advantage of allowing balloon angioplasty and stent insertion in the same procedure (PCI), as well as actual thrombus extraction. Other invasive imaging techniques during invasive angiography such as intravascular ultrasound or optical coherence tomography performed inside the coronary artery can allow visualisation of the plaque structure and aid diagnosis and treatment. However, coronary angiography is an invasive procedure that carries a low risk of significant complications, and there is also a low risk from the radiation received (much lower than the dose received during a nuclear scan or CT angiogram). Coronary angiography is usually reserved for guiding or giving treatment when the diagnosis of ACS is clear or when other non-invasive tests are indeterminate or indicate coronary disease. In patients with definite ACS it is the primary investigation.

Echocardiography

Ultrasound may be useful in the diagnosis of ACS where the ECG is near normal. Abnormalities of wall motion or of left ventricular function may be detected, although this will not tell if these signs are new or longstanding. However, with a good history of chest pain, ultrasound may give increased confidence of new injury before biochemical markers are available (Atar *et al.*, 2004).

Computed tomographic angiography

Computed tomographic (CT) coronary angiography has now developed to be able to image the coronary arteries. It is non-invasive but gives relatively high doses of radiation. Views can be limited when there is calcification within the arteries. Traditional coronary angiography has advantages when ACS is definite, as it the means by which treatment can be given.

CT angiography has been limited until recently by the speed at which the radiation detector array can circle the patient. In effect, it was impossible to image the heart within a single heartbeat. Electron-beam CT angiography answered this problem by moving the X-ray beam, rather than the detectors; however, the cost of this equipment and its limited use means it is not widely available. Recently, more modern CT scanners with arrays of several hundred detectors have brought this imaging modality to the Emergency Department (Vanhoenacker *et al.*, 2007). While this technique allows three-dimensional views of the heart and coronary arteries to be reconstructed, it does not readily allow the interventional techniques of coronary angiography and is not yet widely used in the UK.

Summary

In summary, acute coronary syndromes are diagnosed from the patient's history and presentation, the presence of changes in their ECG and their cardiac troponin level. Practically, treatment is initiated on the first two factors, as the troponin level may not be elevated until 12 hours after the event. Assessment of the patient should be focused and rapid, and carried out in an area where they can be resuscitated if necessary. The presence or absence of changes in the ECG and the troponin level allows the ACS to be categorised and will form part of the patient's risk stratification. Risk stratification allows those patients who are most likely to benefit to receive treatments such as invasive imaging and revascularisation.

References

Antman E, Cohen M, Bernink P and McCabe CH (2000) The TIMI risk score for unstable angina/non-ST elevation MI: a method for prognostication and therapeutic decision making. *Journal of the American Medical Association* **284**(7): 835-42.

Arntz H, Bossaert L and Gerasimos SF (2005) European Resuscitation Council guidelines for resuscitation 2005. Section 5. Initial management of acute coronary syndromes. *Resuscitation* **67**(S1): S87-S96.

Atar S, Feldman A, Darawshe A, Siegel RJ and Rosenfeld T (2004) Utility and diagnostic accuracy of hand-carried ultrasound for emergency room evaluation of chest pain. *American Journal of Cardiology* **94**: 408-9.

Culic V (2002) Symptom presentation of acute myocardial infarction: influence of sex, age, and risk factors. *American Heart Journal* **144**(6): 1012-17.

Ebell MH, Flewelling D and Flynn CA (2000) A systematic review of troponin T and I for diagnosing acute myocardial infarction. *Journal of Family Practice* **49**: 550-6.

Fox KAA, Poole-Wilson P, Clayton TC, Henderson RA, Shaw TR and Wheatley DJ (2005) 5-Year outcome of an interventional strategy in non-ST-elevation acute coronary syndrome. *Lancet* **366**(9489): 914-20.

Fox KAA, Birkhead J, Wilcox R, Knight C and Barth J (2004) British Cardiac Society Working Group on the definition of myocardial infarction. *Heart* **90**: 603-9.

Granger CB, Goldberg RJ, Dabbous O *et al.* (2003) Predictors of hospital mortality in the global registry of acute cardiac events. *Archives of Internal Medicine* **163**: 2345-53.

Sleight P (1981) Cardiac vomiting. *British Heart Journal* **46**: 5-7.

Thygesen K, Alpert JS and White HD (2007) Universal definition of myocardial infarction. *European Heart Journal* **28**: 2525-38.

Van de Werf F, Ardissino D, Betriu A *et al.* (2003) Management of acute myocardial infarction in patients presenting with ST-segment elevation. *European Heart Journal* **24**: 28-66.

Vanhoenacker PK, Decramer I, Bladt O, Sarno G, Bevernage C and Wijns W (2007) Detection of non-ST-segment myocardial infarction and unstable angina in the acute setting: meta-analysis of diagnostic performance of multi-detector computed tomographic angiography. *BMC Cardiovascular Disorders* **7**(39). Available at http://biomedcentral.com/1471-2261/7/39

Webb SW, Adgey AA and Pantridge JF (1972) Autonomic disturbance at onset of acute myocardial infarction. *British Medical Journal* **3**: 89-92.

Williamson K, Mattu A, Plautz CU, Binder A and Brady WJ (2006) Electrocardiographic applications of lead aVR. *American Journal of Emergency Medicine* **24**: 864-74.

Other resources

A series of articles on interpreting the ECG has been published in the *British Medical Journal*, the first appeared in April 2002 (volume 324, pages 831-4), with further articles appearing in subsequent weeks. These are short, bite-size articles, but cover ECG analysis in depth.

Web resources

American College of Cardiology, www.acc.org. This has some excellent webcast presentations by experts in their field.

American Heart Association, www.americanheart.org

British Cardiovascular Society, www.bcs.com

European Society for Cardiology, www.escardio.com, has freely downloadable guidelines on a large number of cardiovascular conditions.

GRACE Registry, www.outcomes-umassmed.org/grace/, has a downloadable risk stratification tool, as well as other information on risk stratification

National Institute for Health and Clinical Excellence, www.nice.org.uk

Scottish Inter-collegiate Guidelines Network, www.sign.ac.uk/guidelines/fulltext/93-97/index.html, has expert opinion on best practice in acute coronary syndromes

TIMI risk stratification tool, www.mdcalc.com/timi-risk-score-for-uanstemi

Chapter 5
Unstable Angina

John McGowan

Introduction

Unstable angina forms part of the spectrum of acute coronary syndromes (ACS). In common with ST segment elevation and non-ST segment elevation myocardial infarction, the patient with unstable angina may have unstable plaque and thrombus in their coronary arteries; there is minimal or no myocardial necrosis. However, there are other critical events that may lead to unstable angina and these will be explored in this chapter. The aim of the chapter is to recognise the patient with unstable angina and understand the rationale for treatment and management.

Learning outcomes

At the end of this chapter the reader will be able to:

- describe the presentation of the patient with unstable angina
- describe the assessment of the patient with unstable angina
- discuss the clinical significance of the investigations undertaken to confirm diagnosis
- describe the immediate care priorities of the patient diagnosed with unstable angina
- critically evaluate the ongoing treatment strategies for the patient diagnosed with unstable angina.

Nursing the Cardiac Patient, First Edition. Edited by Melanie Humphreys.
© 2011 Blackwell Publishing Ltd. Published 2011 by Blackwell Publishing Ltd.

Unstable angina in perspective

Pathogenesis

With unstable angina the flow of blood in the coronary arteries is markedly reduced, leading to the patient experiencing pain at rest or on minimal exertion. This difference in symptoms can be explained by the different nature of atherosclerotic plaque in the coronary arteries. The plaque of stable angina is intact but reduces the size of the lumen of the artery, limiting the rate at which blood can flow through it. In contrast, the coronary artery plaque in unstable angina may have ruptured or eroded, exposing the plaque core to blood flow. This core, which includes lipid, vascular smooth muscle cells, lymphocytes and modified macrophages called foam cells, is highly thrombogenic (Falk *et al.*, 1995). Its exposure causes platelet activation, thrombin production and fibrin deposition, resulting in thrombus formation in the artery, markedly reducing the lumen and blood flow. In addition, plaque content and small emboli from the thrombus may migrate, occluding smaller vessels distal to the rupture. It is the presence of thrombus in the artery that makes unstable angina an ACS. However, there are other critical events that may lead to unstable angina; it may present as troponin-negative and may arise because a coronary stenosis has grown so tight that it limits the blood supply, or in multi-vessel coronary disease the worsening of a single lesion can disrupt the balance of a potentially critical blood supply.

The trigger for the rupture or erosion of plaque in unstable angina is unclear. The relative contributions of plaque contents to its stability and also inflammatory processes have been proposed as causes. The inflammatory marker C-reactive protein may be elevated in unstable angina. While a widespread, large quantity of plaques can lead to unstable angina, it is clear that atherosclerotic plaque is subject to dynamic processes and that plaque rupture and erosion occur without the patient suffering pain, often many times. Indeed, one study has demonstrated that a significant number of people without symptoms have evidence of plaque rupture and erosion in their coronary arteries (Falk *et al.*, 1995). The finding that plaque which ruptures may not be causing a flow-limiting stenosis prior to rupture suggests the quality, rather than quantity, of the plaque is more important (Braganza and Bennett, 2001).

The pain of unstable angina arises from myocardium that is ischaemic, i.e. there is insufficient oxygen to meet tissue demands. In stable angina this may be due to increased tissue demand, for example on exercise, with blood flow limited by atheroma.

Uniqueness of unstable angina

Unlike the other acute coronary syndromes, unstable angina is diagnosed from the patient's history and presentation plus the absence, rather than presence, of changes in the 12-lead ECG and lack of elevated biochemical markers. This definition of unstable angina follows that of the British Cardiovascular Society and of the joint European Society for Cardiology/ American College of Cardiology definitions, which are the nature of the patient's symptoms, with evidence of cardiac disease, no ECG evidence of myocardial infarction and negative troponins (SIGN, 2007).

Despite the absence of evidence of myocytes necrosis in these patients, they are at a high risk of death. One study demonstrated mortality at 30 days after admission of 4.5% and 8.6% at six months after admission (Das et al., 2006). Their care is best managed by a cardiology service, and risk stratification should be carried out using a tool such as the GRACE score (Granger et al., 2003).

Presentation

The most common presenting symptom of unstable angina is chest pain, which is often described as a tight or heavy pain. There may be associated pain in the arms, more commonly the left arm, and the throat or jaw. The pain of unstable angina differs from the pain of stable angina in that either:

- the pain lasts more than 20 minutes at rest
- the patient has developed new angina pain that severely limits mild physical activity, such as walking or climbing stairs or which occurs at rest (Campeau, 1976)
- the patient with stable angina now experiences anginal pain that severely limits mild physical activity, such as walking or climbing stairs or which occurs at rest, this is commonly described as crescendo angina
- the patient has developed angina pain following a myocardial infarction (Bassand et al., 2007).

Less frequently, the presenting symptoms of unstable angina include breathlessness, palpitations, epigastric discomfort, shoulder or neck pain and syncope. Some patient groups, notably women, diabetics and elderly patients, are more likely to describe atypical symptoms (Culic, 2002). Patients with dementia may have difficulty expressing their symptoms and will often describe atypical symptoms (Canto et al., 2002).

Assessment

Assessment of the patient with a suspected acute coronary event will comprise:

- rapid ABCDE evaluation and the recording of vital signs
- taking a focused patient history
- investigations including a 12-lead ECG
- routine baseline blood chemistry.

The history taken from the patient should be rapid and focused (*see* Chapter 3 for comprehensive discussion). It should allow the nurse to assess the likelihood of the patient having an ACS and their potential risk of sudden deterioration. Some of the questions that must be asked will include the following.

- Did the patient experience chest pain?
- When did the symptoms begin?
- How long did the chest pain last?
- Are there any other symptoms associated with it?
- Have there been any previous episodes of chest pain?
- Has the patient had any previous illnesses or surgery, for example diabetes or cardiac surgery?
- Does the patient have any allergies?
- What drugs is the patient is taking, prescribed and non-prescribed, including smoking history?
- Is there any family history of heart disease?

Investigations

A 12-lead ECG should be performed as soon as possible, both to detect any changes and to provide a baseline against which any subsequent ECGs can be compared. It is worth noting that the initial ECG in these patients may be grossly normal. In the event of the patient experiencing further chest pain or worsening symptoms, this investigation should be repeated. See Figure 5.1.

In some cases, this investigation will be repeated at half-hourly intervals, allowing early detection of changes of myocardial infarction and resolution of acute ischaemic changes.

Continuous 12-lead ST segment monitoring, allowing detection of transient changes in these can be used if available (Bassand *et al.*, 2007), but otherwise standard cardiac monitoring should be commenced.

Patients presenting with a history suggestive of unstable angina should not be discharged home on the basis of a normal ECG, unless their history and investigation results have been reviewed by a senior member of medical staff. Several studies have noted alarmingly high numbers of patients with chest pain discharged from Emergency Departments who were subsequently found to have unstable angina or myocardial infarction (Bassand *et al.*, 2007). However, diagnosis of unstable angina does not depend on the patient having ECG changes.

Venous blood should be sent for urea and electrolytes, liver function tests, troponin, full blood count, glucose and C-reactive protein. The patient's potassium should be normalised and creatinine level will be used in risk stratification. Although creatinine is utilised rarely as a risk tool, it has been reported that patients with elevated creatinine will have a higher risk stratification score (Granger *et al.*, 2003).

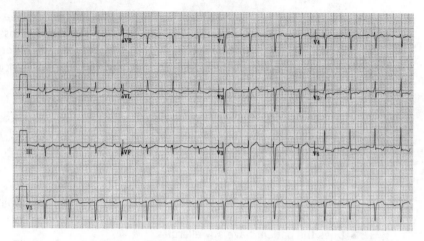

Figure 5.1 The 12-lead ECG of a 71-year-old man with increasing anginal pain, culminating in 40 minutes of chest pain, at rest, eased by morphine. The rhythm is sinus, there is T wave inversion in leads I, aVL, V_5 and V_6, with ST segment depression in leads II, III, aVF, V_5 and V_6. He was diagnosed as having an acute coronary syndrome, unstable angina and treated with oxygen, nitrate, aspirin, clopidogrel and low molecular weight heparin. His troponin I at 12 hours was 0.01 ng/l, which the lab stated showed no evidence of myocardial necrosis. He had no further pain and underwent balloon angioplasty and insertion of a stent three days after admission and was subsequently discharged home.

Anaemia reduces the capacity of the blood to carry oxygen and may exacerbate the symptoms of unstable angina. Elevated blood glucose should be controlled with insulin if necessary. Elevated C-reactive protein is known to be predictive of a higher risk of death or myocardial infarction in the six months after the presenting event (Heeschen et al., 2000). An arterial blood gas sample may be taken if the patient is breathless or has a low oxygen saturation on oximetry. Oxygen may be administered even with normal saturation. A portable chest X-ray should be requested to exclude other pathology. Echocardiography should be carried out to assess left ventricular function and to detect structural or wall motion abnormalities.

Treatment strategies

The management of unstable angina is aimed at reducing oxygen demand and prevention of further thrombus formation or proliferation. Despite the presence of clot in the coronary artery, no benefit has been demonstrated from the use of fibrinolytics in unstable angina.

The five main categories of the immediate management of unstable angina are:

- rest and analgesia
- anti-ischaemic therapy

- anti-platelet therapy
- anticoagulants
- plaque stabilisation.

Rest and analgesia

As the symptoms of unstable angina are caused by a reduced oxygen supply to the myocardium, there is a certain logic in limiting the amount of oxygen consumed in other tissues by preventing the patient from exercising. On a practical note, having the patient confined to bed allows them to be closely observed and their vital signs, including their heart rhythm, to be monitored. All patients with acute coronary syndromes should be treated in a high dependency care area, with resuscitation equipment and qualified staff trained in its use should resuscitation to be required.

Patients with unstable angina will usually require analgesia, for example opiates such as morphine or diamorphine. These should be administered intravenously. An anti-emetic may also be administered with these.

Anti-ischaemic therapy

These treatments are targeted at reducing the oxygen consumption of the myocardium by reducing its work.

Nitrates, such as glyceryl trinitrate (GTN), may be given by sublingual spray, by buccally absorbed tablets or by continuous intravenous infusion. These reduce cardiac work by reducing preload and left ventricular end diastolic pressure. They also cause systemic vasodilation and may improve blood flow in the coronary arteries by dilating these. Patients on nitrate infusions should have their blood pressure closely monitored as this vasodilation can cause hypotension.

Beta-blockers prevent noradrenaline binding to beta adrenoceptors in sympathetic neurons and reduce oxygen consumption, in the main by slowing the heart rate. They may worsen asthma, heart failure and diabetes, and should be used cautiously where patients have any of these. Beta-blockers are contraindicated in patients with known bradycardia or heart block.

Calcium channel blockers reduce oxygen consumption in a similar manner to nitrates, by causing vasodilation. Some will also cause a slight reduction in heart rate. These drugs are useful where symptoms are exacerbated by coronary artery spasm (Bassand et al., 2007). Rate-slowing calcium channel blockers such as diltiazem or verapamil vasodilate and reduce the heart rate, and can be effective therapies in patients who have contraindications to beta-blockers. They should not be used in the presence of bradycardias, heart block or heart failure.

Anti-platelet therapy

Thrombus is a matrix formed by activated platelets and fibrin strands. The aim of anti-platelet and anticoagulant therapy is to prevent extension and

Table 5.1 Summary of actions of anticoagulant and anti-platelet drugs

Drug	Mode of action
Aspirin	Low dose inhibits platelet activation by blocking thromboxane α_2 synthesis
Clopidogrel	Prevents ADP-dependent activation of glycoprotein IIb/IIIa receptors
Abciximab Eptifibatide Tirofiban	Bind to glycoprotein IIb/IIIa receptors competing with fibrinogen, reducing bonds to adjacent platelets
Heparin Fondaparinux	Inhibit factor Xa and so reduce fibrin production

reduce the size of existing thrombus, as well as preventing new thrombus from being formed.

Platelets are activated by a number of pathways, which means that simply blocking one pathway will not prevent activation. Anti-platelet drugs used in unstable angina therefore target both platelet activation and the receptors that bind fibrinogen to link adjacent platelets, the glycoprotein IIb/IIIa receptors (Table 5.1).

Platelet activation is mediated by a balance between two compounds. Thromboxane α_2, which promotes aggregation, and prostacyclin, which inhibits aggregation. Low-dose aspirin prevents synthesis of thromboxane α_2; at higher doses prostacyclin is also inhibited (Rang et al., 2001). A number of large trials have shown the benefit of low-dose aspirin in ACS (Collins et al., 1997). Patients with unstable angina should have aspirin 300 mg, either chewed or crushed, as soon as possible, and 75–150 mg daily thereafter (Patrono et al., 2004). Buccal absorption of the crushed or chewed aspirin allows rapid anti-platelet activity. The main contraindications to aspirin are allergy and gastrointestinal bleeding.

The glycoprotein IIb/IIIa receptors that allow platelets to bind to each other are activated by ADP. Clopidogrel (Plavix), is one example, which inhibits this ADP-dependent activation, reducing the ability of platelets to clump together. Patients with unstable angina should have clopidogrel 300 mg orally as soon as possible and 75 mg daily, for up to 12 months (Bassand et al., 2007); higher loading doses of 600 mg are used it the patient is going for urgent angiography. The main contraindication to clopidogrel is bleeding. Caution is needed with non-steroidal anti-inflammatory drugs as their metabolism may be slowed.

Anticoagulant therapy

Heparin and the synthetic pentasaccharide fondaparinux (Arixtra) inhibit the binding of factor Xa in the blood, preventing prothrombin being converted to thrombin in the early part of the coagulation cascade, which results in the formation of fibrin. Platelets produce factor Xa, which is protected from the actions of unfractionated heparin, and platelet factor 4, which neutralises unfractionated heparin. Low molecular weight heparin is not modified by this platelet activity (Rang *et al.*, 2001). In addition, low molecular weight heparin given subcutaneously does not need to be closely monitored by blood sampling. Patients with unstable angina should commence anticoagulation with low molecular weight heparin as soon as possible. Bivalirudan (Angiomax), which acts as a direct thrombin inhibitor may also be added.

Plaque stabilisation

Given that unstable angina is a disease of unstable plaque in the coronary arteries, there has been interest in recent years in ways to stabilise this. Statins, (HMG co-enzyme A reductase inhibitors) are mainstay drugs in primary and secondary prevention of coronary heart disease, acting to reduce low-density lipoprotein cholesterol, and have been demonstrated to reduce the incidence of acute cardiovascular events. The finding at angiography that despite lipid lowering with statins, in most cases established plaques do not shrink in size, together with animal models which suggest that statins alter the components of plaque, has led to the view that these drugs act, in part, by reducing the propensity of plaque to rupture or erode (Braganza and Bennett, 2001); there has been exception of late with some evidence suggesting that atorvastatin does actually cause plaque regression (Yonemura *et al.*, 2005). Whether this is by anti-inflammatory action or changing the proportions of the constituents of plaque is unclear. Patients with unstable angina should receive lipid reduction treatment with statins as early as possible in their admission.

Angiotensin-converting enzyme inhibitors such as ramipril or enalapril are also thought to have an anti-atherosclerotic effect and have been shown to reduce adverse events in patients with stable coronary heart disease. There has been a recent recommendation that these drugs should be prescribed to patients with unstable disease, including unstable angina (Bassand *et al.*, 2007; HOPE, 2000).

Revascularisation

Patients with no ECG changes during pain who are troponin-negative need consideration of all causes of chest pain, including coronary disease. Non-invasive assessment for low-risk patients with stress testing with plain exercise, nuclear cardiology or stress echocardiography can be used to risk stratify low-risk patients. High-risk patients or patients who have positive non-invasive assessment should have angiography with a view to revascularisation prior to discharge (*see* Chapter 6).

Summary

Unstable angina is part of the spectrum of acute coronary syndromes and is a clinical syndrome caused by plaque rupture and erosion with thrombus formation in the coronary arteries, or by increasing narrowing of the stenosis. It carries significant mortality at both at 30 days and at six months after the acute event. Diagnosis is made on a patient history of prolonged chest pain, new chest pain on minimal exercise, crescendo pain or pain following previous myocardial infarction. The ECG will have no new signs of myocardial infarction and the patient's troponin level will be normal.

Patients' risk profiles should be evaluated, and all causes of chest pain should be considered in patients with normal ECGs and negative troponins. Low-risk patients can be considered for non-invasive assessment prior to discharge. High-risk patients or patients with positive non-invasive tests should have inpatient angiography to elucidate the right revascularisation strategy.

References

Bassand JP, Hamm CW, Ardissino D et al. (2007) Guidelines for the diagnosis and treatment of non-ST-segment elevation acute coronary syndromes. European Heart Journal 28(13): 1598-660.

Braganza DM and Bennett MR (2001) New insights into atherosclerotic plaque rupture. Postgraduate Medical Journal 77: 94-8.

Campeau L (1976) Grading of angina pectoris. Circulation 54: 522-3.

Canto JG, Finscher C, Kiefe CI et al. (2002) Atypical presentations among Medicare benificiaries with unstable angina pectoris. American Journal of Cardiology 90: 248-53.

Collins R, Peto R, Baigent C and Sleight P (1997) Aspirin, heparin and fibrinolytic therapy in suspected acute myocardial infarction. New England Journal of Medicine 336(12): 847-60.

Culic V (2002) Symptom presentation of acute myocardial infarction: influence of sex, age, and risk factors. American Heart Journal 144(6): 1012-17.

Das R, Kilcullen N, Morrell C, Robinson MB, Barth JH and Hall AS (2006) The British Cardiac Society Working Group definition of myocardial infarction: implications for practice. Heart 92: 21-6.

Falk E, Prediman KS and Fuster V (1995) Coronary plaque disruption. Circulation 92: 657-71.

Granger CB, Goldberg RJ, Dabbous O et al. (2003) Predictors of hospital mortality in the global registry of acute cardiac events. Archives of Internal Medicine 163: 2345-53.

Heeschen C, Hamm CW, Bruemmer J and Simoons ML (2000) Predictive value of C-reactive protein and troponin T in patients with unstable angina: a comparative analysis. Journal of the American College of Cardiology 35: 1535-42.

The HOPE Study (Heart Outcomes Prevention Evaluation) (2000) Journal of Renin Angiotensin Aldosterone System 1(1): 18-20.

Patrono C, Bachman F, Baigent et al. (2004) Expert consensus document on the use of antiplatelet agents. European Heart Journal 25: 166-81.

Rang HP, Dale MM and Ritter JM (2001) Pharmacology (4e). Edinburgh, Harcourt.

Scottish Intercollegiate Guidelines Network (SIGN) (2007) *SIGN 93: Acute Coronary Syndromes*. Available at www.sign.ac.uk

Yonemura A, Momiyama Y, Fayad Z *et al*. (2005) Effect of lipid-lowering therapy with atorvastatin on atherosclerotic aortic plaques detected by noninvasive magnetic resonance imaging. *Journal of the American College of Cardiology* **45**(5): 733-42.

Chapter 6

Non-ST Segment Elevation Myocardial Infarction

Melanie Humphreys

Introduction

Cardiovascular diseases exert a huge burden on individuals and society, with coronary heart disease (CHD) the single most common cause of death in the UK and other developed countries (British Heart Foundation, 2009). All cardiac events are particularly distressing and frightening, not only for patients but also for relatives. Activity, levels of anxiety, speed of onset and previous experience may influence patients' perception of its severity. This chapter continues within the acute coronary syndrome (ACS) theme, moving the focus to the patient with a non-ST segment elevation myocardial infarction (NSTEMI). Distinguishing a NSTEMI from unstable angina and ST segment elevation myocardial infarction (STEMI) is important; the practitioner will need a good understanding of assessment, diagnosis, treatment and management strategies, all of which are essential to reducing the patient risk. Through a structured approach of assessment, initiating investigations, treatment and delivering appropriate care, timely interventions will be afforded. The aim of this chapter is to understand the management of NSTEMI within an evidence-based framework.

Learning outcomes

At the end of this chapter the reader will be able to:

- describe the initial presentation and assessment of the patient presenting with a NSTEMI
- discuss the concept of NSTEMI and detail the treatment and care priorities of these patients
- critically discuss the ongoing care strategies for the patient who has experienced a NSTEMI.

Nursing the Cardiac Patient, First Edition. Edited by Melanie Humphreys.
© 2011 Blackwell Publishing Ltd. Published 2011 by Blackwell Publishing Ltd.

Non-ST segment elevation myocardial infarction in perspective

Non-ST segment elevation myocardial infarction is one of the three types of ACS, and like all ACS, NSTEMI should be considered a medical emergency. NSTEMI is identical to unstable angina except for one thing. In NSTEMI, cardiac enzyme blood tests are abnormal, indicating that at least some actual cell damage is occurring to heart muscle cells. The patient with NSTEMI will be experiencing the same critical events that led to disruption in the cardiac blood supply, which include unstable plaque and thrombus in their coronary arteries and critical coronary stenosis that is limiting the blood supply; in multi-vessel coronary disease, the worsening of a single lesion can disrupt the balance of a potentially critical blood supply.

Fundamentally, in every other way NSTEMI and unstable angina are identical. They both indicate a partial blockage of the artery, and that the myocardium supplied by that artery is in grave danger of sustaining irreversible damage. In other words, the imminent risk of a STEMI, with irreversible ischaemia and necrosis to the myocardium, is high in both NSTEMI and unstable angina.

Many cardiac arrests are caused by underlying coronary artery disease and occur in the context of an ACS (Resuscitation Council, 2010). It is therefore essential that practitioners understand the basis of ACS and implement appropriate treatment strategies. This is guided initially be the patient's symptoms and ECG changes (*see* Chapter 4). Treatment should not be delayed to await the appearance of biochemical markers that may not be detectable for several hours after the onset of symptoms (Edwards and Pitcher, 2005). The aim for all patients is universal: to alleviate symptoms, resuscitate if necessary and provide prompt and effective restoration or protection of coronary blood flow to relieve ischaemia and prevent further myocardial damage; ultimately this will reduce the risk of cardiac arrest and death.

Causes

Pathogenesis

The common underlying causative mechanism is sudden fissuring, erosion or rupture of the cap of an atherosclerotic plaque in a coronary artery. Subendothelial collagen becomes exposed and promotes platelet adhesion, aggregation and activation. A surrounding fibrin-rich thrombus develops around the platelets and is accompanied by a complex set of reactions including vasoconstriction, inflammation and micro-embolism (Edwards and Pitcher, 2005). The result is reduced coronary arterial blood flow, but the pathological and clinical consequences are variable, depending on whether occlusion of the coronary artery is partial or total, the degree of collateral blood flow to the affected myocardium and the mass of myocardium affected (Figure 6.1).

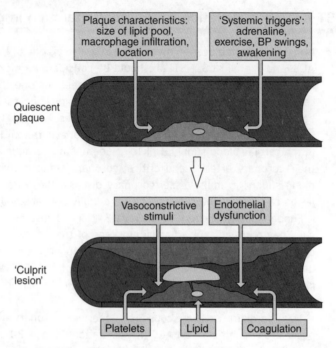

Figure 6.1 Unstable plaque "culprit lesion". From Jevon P, Humphreys M and Ewens B (2009) *Nursing Medical Emergency Patients*. Reproduced with permission from John Wiley & Sons.

Uniqueness of NSTEMI

The diagnosis of NSTEMI is based on a history of acute cardiac ischaemia in the absence of ST segment elevation. In NSTEMI it is common for the ruptured atherosclerotic plaque to have caused incomplete coronary artery occlusion. Alternatively, the myocardium may have been protected by good collateral flow or may have a relatively low oxygen demand. This different underlying situation is the basis for the different effectiveness of and approaches to treatment from those used in STEMI (*see* Chapter 7).

The signs and symptoms of NSTEMI include:

- chest pain (Figure 6.2):
  - characteristic, excruciating, "crushing", "throbbing", type of pain, retrosternal, radiates to the left shoulder, left ulnar part of arm, lower jaw, neck, abdomen to the umbilicus
  - lasts for longer time than anginal pain - usually >30 minutes
  - may have onset at rest - unlike stable angina
  - not relieved by rest or nitro-glycerine
  - 15-20% of infarcts are painless - especially in patients with diabetes and in the elderly - in these cases it may present as acute onset of breathlessness and signs of pulmonary oedema (*see* Chapter 7)
- shortness of breath

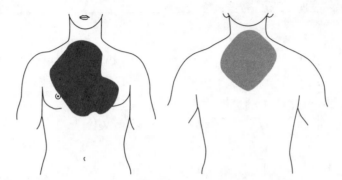

Figure 6.2 Typical chest pain distribution in ACS – front and back. From Jevon P, Humphreys M and Ewens B (2009) *Nursing Medical Emergency Patients*. Reproduced with permission from John Wiley & Sons.

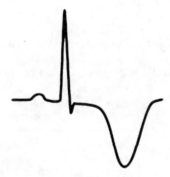

Figure 6.3 T wave inversion.

- nausea
- vomiting
- diaphoresis (sweating)
- palpitations
- anxiety or sense of impending doom
- a feeling of being acutely ill
- non-specific ECG changes – ST segment depression/T wave inversion (*see* Figures 6.3 and 6.4)
- raised troponin levels (amount released reflects extent of myocardial damage).

Myocardial ischaemia may give rise to T wave inversion, but it should be remembered that inverted T waves are normal in leads III, aVR and V_1 in association with a predominantly negative QRS complex. T waves that are deep and symmetrically inverted (arrowhead) strongly suggest myocardial ischaemia.

The treatment of NSTEMI differs in some respect from the treatment of STEMI as the focus here is dictated largely by assessment of risk.

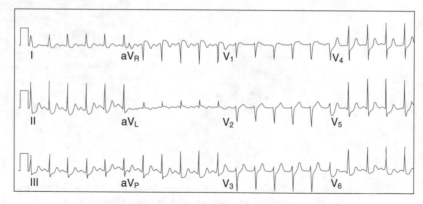

Figure 6.4 12-lead ECG demonstrating ST segment depression in leads I, II, III, aVF, V_4-V_6. From Jevon P, Humphreys M and Ewens B (2009) *Nursing Medical Emergency Patients*. Reproduced with permission from John Wiley & Sons.

Table 6.1 Spectrum of acute coronary syndrome

	ACS with unstable angina	ACS with myocyte necrosis (NSTEMI)	ACS with clinical myocardial infarction (STEMI)
Marker	Troponin (Tn) and CK-MB undetectable	Troponin elevated Tn T < 1.0 ng/ml	Tn T > 1.0 ng/ml +/- ↑CK-MB
ECG	ST↓ or T↓ Transient ST↑ Normal	ST↓ or T↓ Transient ST↑ Normal	ST↑ or ST↓ or T inversion May evolve Q waves
Risk of death	5-8%	8-12%	12-15%
Pathology	Plaque disruption, intra-coronary thrombus, micro-emboli Partial coronary occlusion -------------- Complete occlusion		
LV function	No measurable dysfunction ----- systolic dysfunction, LV dilation		

Adapted from the British Cardiac Society (2004).

Diagnosis

NSTEMI is only one of the many potential causes of chest pain; however, it is safer to treat the patient as if it is cardiac in origin until proven otherwise (Table 6.1).

Initial examination will include (*see* Chapters 3 and 4 for a fuller description) the following.

- Reported history of acute cardiac ischaemia:
  - abrupt new onset of severe ischaemic chest pain, deterioration of previously stable angina or crescendo anginal symptoms in frequency and severity.
- 12-lead ECG.
- Blood tests (in particular serum cardiac markers such as troponin I/T and/ or CK-MB, but also including urea and electrolytes, random glucose, random cholesterol and full blood count).
- Chest X-ray (portable – only if the cause is not thought to be cardiac; it is not appropriate to send the patient to the X-ray department in the acute situation).

These will be evaluated in conjunction with a rapid history and examination focusing primarily on the cardiovascular system (Connaughton, 2001) and a diagnosis made.

Cardiac enzymes

NSTEMI belongs to the single clinical entity pathway that represents the entire clinical spectrum for ACS; the clinical approach focuses on risk stratification, in which cardiac markers have assumed a central role (American College of Cardiology [ACC; Braunwald *et al.*, 2000], European Society of Cardiology [ESC; 2000] and British Cardiac Society [Fox *et al.*, 2004]) (*see* Table 6.2).

The best cardiac marker for each case depends on the time from onset of symptoms; the earliest markers are myoglobin and CK-MB isoforms (1-4 h). CK-MB and troponins are ideal in the intermediate period of 6-24 h. The troponins are recommended for elevation in patients who present more than 24 hours after symptom onset (discussed more fully in Chapter 4).

There are other non-cardiac conditions that troponins may be raised (i.e. renal failure, heart failure, etc.); therefore, the clinical context is very important.

Table 6.2 Table of cardiac markers in response to myocardial injury

Serum markers of myocardial injury	Detected (h)	Peak (h)	Falls (h)	Normal value
Myoglobin	1-3	1-8	12-18	<1
CK-MB Isoforms	1-6	4-8	12-48	<1
Troponin complex	3-6	10-24	TnI: 5-9 days TnT: 7-14 days	<0.4 <0.01 >0.1 (indicative of an MI)

> **Box 6.1 TIMI (thrombolysis in myocardial infarction) risk score for unstable angina/non-ST-segment elevation myocardial infarction**
>
> If present, each of the following contributes +1 to the overall score.
>
> - Score >4 indicates high-risk non-ST-segment elevation ACS.
> - Age ≥65 years.
> - At least three risk factors for coronary artery disease: male sex, hyperlipidaemia, hypertension, smoking, diabetes mellitus, family history of premature coronary disease.
> - Previous coronary stenosis ≥50 per cent.
> - ST-segment elevation or depression at presentation.
> - Two or more anginal events in the past 24 hours.
> - Aspirin use in the past 7 days.
> - Elevated serum cardiac biomarkers.
>
> (Antman *et al.*, 2000)

Treatment of NSTEMI

If the ECG does not show ST segment elevation, the term NSTEMI is applied. The accepted management of NSTEMI is empirical and initial treatment is guided by risk assessment (Gibler *et al.*, 2005). Patients are stratified by haemodynamic, biochemical and medical factors, into high, intermediate and low risk groups (European Society of Cardiology, 2002), it is risk status which drives pharmacological treatments and the timing of further interventional procedures (Antman *et al.*, 2000; *see* Box 6.1).

Treatment for patients with NSTEMI typically consists of the following.

Pain relief

Effective pain relief is a priority and can be provided before a 12-lead ECG is recorded (Erhardt *et al.*, 2002).

- Intravenous (IV) morphine/diamorphine is the preferred agent (which may be directed by local policy) and titrated according to response until all pain has dissipated.
- Consider a suitable antiemetic, e.g. metoclopramide or cyclizine.

Anti-platelet agents

Anti-platelet agents work on various steps of the platelet aggregation pathway to prevent clot formation.

- Aspirin 300 mg (then 75-150 mg daily); should be administered early in all ACS unless absolutely contraindicated (ISIS-2, 1988).
- Platelet ADP receptor antagonist such as clopidogrel or prasugrel. (Resuscitation Council, 2010; NICE, 2004; CURE, 2001).
- Glycoprotein IIb/IIIa inhibitors are recommended as part of initial management of NSTEMI in those at high risk of STEMI or death (NICE, 2002a).

Anti-thrombin agents

The use of heparin is recommended as an essential part of ACS treatment (Bertrand *et al.*, 2002). Heparin blocks thrombin production, and can reduce thrombus formation and facilitate resolution.

- Low molecular weight heparin subcutaneously (e.g. enoxaparin 3-6 days) (ASSENT, 2001).

Anti-ischaemic therapies

Anti-ischaemic therapies decrease myocardial oxygen use by decreasing heart rate, lowering blood pressure or decreasing left ventricular contractility or induce vasodilatation. They can also provide pain relief when ischaemia is the cause of pain (Erhardt *et al.*, 2002; NICE, 2002b).

- Nitrates (IV if high risk).
- Beta-blockers (IV if high risk).
- Rate slowing calcium channel blockers such as verapamil or diltiazem if the heart rate is high. (for recurrent ischaemia, particularly if beta-blockers are contraindicated).

Once the patient's condition is stabilised, the focus of management shifts to preventing further cardiac events. This involves treatments to prevent future plaque rupture and thrombus formation. Blood pressure control should be optimised and lipid-lowering therapy initiated.

The following medications have been shown to reduce the recurrence of cardiovascular events and should be used in secondary prevention regimens (Bertrand *et al.*, 2002).

- Aspirin (75 mg/day).
- Clopidogrel (75 mg/day for 12 months).
- Angiotensin-converting enzyme inhibitors (ACE).
- Beta-blockers (bisoprolol 5 mg; atenolol 50 mg; metoprolol 50 mg).
- Rate slowing calcium channel blockers such as verapamil or diltiazem if the heart rate is high and beta-blockers are contraindicated.
- Long acting oral nitrate (e.g. ISMN or ISDN).
- Statins (HMG-CoA reductase inhibitors).

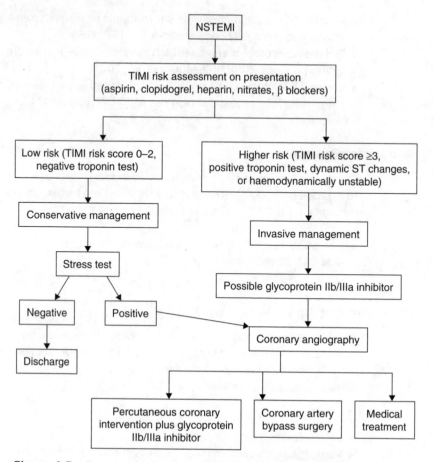

Figure 6.5 An example summary of the treatment for NSTEMI.

Cardiac troponins are measured 12 hours after onset of the pain (see above and Chapters 3 and 4). If this is positive, coronary angiography is typically performed on an urgent basis as this is highly predictive of a heart attack in the near future. If the troponin is negative, a treadmill exercise test or a thallium scintigram may be requested (Figure 6.5).

If any of the following risk factors are present, early angiography is indicated (Fox, 2004; DH, 2000).

- Elevated troponin levels.
- Prolonged rest angina with ECG changes in more than two leads.
- Pulmonary oedema or hypotension.
- Angina not settling with medical treatment.
- Second presentation of ACS within three months.

Summary

NSTEMI is part of the spectrum of ACS and is a clinical syndrome caused by plaque rupture and erosion with thrombus formation in the coronary arteries or by increasing narrowing of a coronary stenosis. As nurses expand their scope of practice they play an ever more important role in the management and subsequent rehabilitation of patients who present with NSTEMI. This chapter has examined the assessment, diagnosis and priorities of care for this patient group in order to facilitate systematic management, to promote prompt initiation of evidence-based treatments.

References

Antman E, Cohen M, Bernink P and McCabe CH (2000) The TIMI risk score for unstable angina/non-ST elevation MI: a method for prognostication and therapeutic decision making. *Journal of the American Medical Association* **284**(7): 835-42.

ASSENT-3 Investigators (2001) Efficacy and safety of tenecteplase in combination with enoxaparin, abcixmab, or unfractionated heparin; the ASSENT-3 randomised trial in acute myocardial infarction. *Lancet* **358**: 605-13.

Baigent C, Collins R, Appleby P and Parish S (1998) ISIS-2: 10-year survival among patients with suspected acute myocardial infarction in randomised comparison of intravenous streptokinase, oral aspirin, both, or neither. The Bertrand ME, Simoons ML and Fox KA (2002) Management of acute coronary syndromes in patients presenting without persistent ST-segment elevation. *European Heart Journal* **23**(23): 1809-40.

Braunwald E, Antman EM, Beasley JW, Califf RM, Cheitlin MD and Hochman JS (2000) ACC/AHA guidelines for the management of patients with unstable angina and non-ST-segment elevation myocardial infarction: executive summary and recommendations. A report of the American College of Cardiology/American Heart Association task force on practice guidelines (committee on the management of patients with unstable angina). *Circulation* **102**: 1193-209.

British Heart Foundation (2009) Coronary heart disease statistics database. www.heartstats.org

The Clopidogrel in Unstable Angina to Prevent Recurrent Events Trial Investigators (CURE) (2001) Effects of clopidogrel in addition to aspirin in patients with acute coronary syndromes without ST-segment elevation. *New England Journal of Medicine* **345**: 494-502.

Connaughton M (2001) *Evidence-based Coronary Care*. London, Churchill Livingstone.

Department of Health (2000) *National Service Framework for Coronary Heart Disease. Modern Standard and Service Models*. London, Department of Health.

Edwards N and Pitcher D (2005) An overview of acute coronary syndromes. *British Journal of Resuscitation* **4**(1): 6-10.

Erhardt L, Herlitz J and Bossaert L (2002) Task force on the management of chest pain. *European Heart Journal* **23**(15): 1153-76.

Fox KA (2004) Management of acute coronary syndromes: an update. *Heart* **90**(6): 698-706.

Fox KA, Birkhead J, Wilcox R, Knight C and Barth J (2004) British Cardiac Society Working Group on the definition of Myocardial Infarction. *Heart* **90**(6): 603-9.

Gibler WB, Cannon CP and Blomkalns AL (2005) Practical implementation of the guidelines for unstable angina/ non-ST-segment elevation myocardial infarction in the emergency department: a scientific statement from the

American Heart Association Council on Clinical Cardiology (Subcommittee on Acute Cardiac Care), Council on Cardiovascular Nursing, and Quality of Care and Outcomes Research Interdisciplinary Working Group, in Collaboration with the Society of Chest Pain Centers. *Circulation* **111**(20): 2699-710.

ISIS-2 (1988) Second international study of infarct survival collaborative group. A randomized trial of intravenous streptokinase, oral aspirin, both or neither among 17,187 cases of suspected acute myocardial infarction. *Lancet* **ii**: 349-60.

Joint European Society of Cardiology/American College of Cardiology committee for the redefinition of myocardial infarction (2000) Myocardial infarction redefined - a consensus document. *Journal of American Cardiology* **36**: 959-69.

National Institute for Health and Clinical Excellence (NICE) (2004) *Technology Appraisal Guidance 80. Clopidogrel in the Treatment of Non-ST Segment- elevation Acute Coronary Syndrome*. London, NICE.

National Institute for Health and Clinical Excellence (NICE) (2002a) *Technology Appraisal Guidance 47. Glycoprotein IIb/IIIa Inhibitor Guidance for Acute Coronary Syndromes*. London, NICE.

National Institute for Health and Clinical Excellence (NICE) (2002b) *Technology Appraisal Guidance 52. Guidance on the Use of Drugs for Early thrombolysis in the Treatment of Acute Myocardial Infarction*. London, NICE.

Resuscitation Council (UK) (2010) *Advanced Life Support Provider Manual*, (5e). London, Resuscitation Council (UK).

Task Force on the Management of Acute Coronary Syndromes of the European Society of Cardiology (2002) Management of acute coronary syndromes in patients presenting without persistent ST segment elevation (ESC). *European Heart Journal* **23:** 1809-40.

Chapter 7
ST Segment Elevation Myocardial Infarction

Claire Rushton

Introduction

In the UK, around 146,000 people suffer an acute myocardial infarction (AMI) each year and there are more than 1.4 million people in the UK estimated to have had an MI at any one time (British Heart Foundation, 2008). AMI leads to a high risk of heart failure and potentially fatal cardiac arrhythmias, both during the acute phase and in the months and years following the event. AMI associated with ST elevation on the electrocardiogram (ECG) is commonly caused by coronary artery thrombosis. More than 10% of people suffering ST elevation MI (STEMI) die within 30 days of admission to hospital (MINAP, 2008). A significant proportion of deaths occur before the patient reaches hospital and those that come into contact with health professionals have so far survived a major cardiac assault (Jowett and Thompson, 2007). Rapid reperfusion strategies together with supporting pharmacological intervention can greatly reduce the risk of mortality. Rapid delivery of appropriate treatment demands fast and accurate diagnosis. The aim of this chapter is to offer a coherent systematic approach towards assessment, interpretation and caring for the patient experiencing a STEMI.

Learning outcomes

At the end of this chapter the reader will be able to:

- describe the initial presentation and assessment of the patient admitted with STEMI
- discuss the clinical significance of the investigations undertaken to confirm diagnosis
- describe the immediate care priorities of the patient experiencing STEMI
- critically evaluate the ongoing care management for the patient who has experienced a STEMI
- identify and discuss the clinical significance of infarct regions.

Nursing the Cardiac Patient, First Edition. Edited by Melanie Humphreys.
© 2011 Blackwell Publishing Ltd. Published 2011 by Blackwell Publishing Ltd.

ST segment elevation myocardial infarction in perspective

ST segment elevation myocardial infarction falls towards the end of the clinical spectrum of acute coronary syndrome. STEMI is defined by myocardial necrosis consistent with myocardial ischaemia indicated by persistent ST segment rise. Patients presenting with STEMI may go on to develop Q waves on their ECG and show a rise in biomarkers indicative of cardiac necrosis (European Society of Cardiology, 2008; Thygesen *et al.*, 2007). This finding will be determined by the speed of reperfusion and resultant myocardial necrosis.

Pathogenesis

Myocardial infarction is cardiac necrosis caused by a cessation of blood flow to the myocardium. This is usually the result of a blockage to one of the major epicardial coronary arteries supplying the myocardium with oxygenated blood (Figure 7.1). Commonly the blockage is caused by a blood clot (thrombus) that forms over a ruptured atherosclerotic plaque. When a vulnerable atherosclerotic plaque ruptures, a chain of events occurs resulting in coronary artery occlusion and a medical emergency (Figure 7.2). If the thrombus fully occludes the coronary artery then STEMI will occur (Moser and Riegal, 2008). Other less common causes of STEMI include coronary artery spasm, coronary dissection, coronary embolism and pericardiac interventions. Anaemia, arrhythmias, hypertension and hypotension can also lead to myocardial injury (Thygesen *et al.*, 2007).

When the blood flow to the myocardium deteriorates, myocardial oxygen demands exceed those of supply and the myocardial cells begin an immedi-

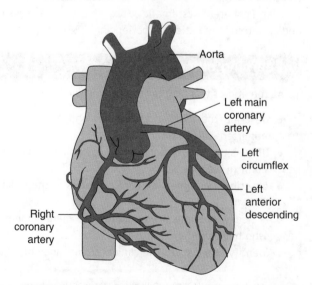

Figure 7.1 Diagrammatic representation of the coronary arteries.

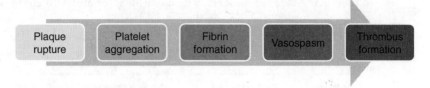

Figure 7.2 Chain of events following the rupture of a vulnerable atherosclerotic plaque.

ate process of demise. Within seconds, systolic contraction stops in the affected area. Following a brief period of ischaemia the myocardium will become injured. During this phase the effected myocardial cells cannot function, but with rapid treatment could be salvaged. Finally, after 15–30 minutes of loss of blood flow the myocardium will begin to infarct and the damage at this stage is irreversible (Conover, 2003) (*see* Table 7.1). Spreading from subendocardium to subepicardium, the time for full-thickness necrosis will be dependent on any collateral blood supply to the affected area (European Society of Cardiology, 2008).

Rapid assessment, diagnosis and treatment in this patient group are essential in order to re-establish perfusion to the myocardium thus minimising infarct size and preserving myocardial function.

Presenting features

Patients suffering from STEMI will present in a variety of ways depending on:

- the size and location of the infarct
- the degree of chest pain experienced
- the response of the autonomic nervous system to injury
- the patient's co-morbidities and previous experience.

Generally patients will present with:

- chest pain
- nausea and possible vomiting
- dyspnoea (breathlessness)
- anxiety or a feeling of "impending doom"
- diaphoresis (sweating)
- pallor.

Most of the common presenting symptoms will result from the activation of the autonomic nervous system in response to injury, pain and anxiety. Sympathetic nervous response can lead to peripheral vasoconstriction causing the patient to look pale, and feel cool and clammy. As blood is moved

Table 7.1 Stages of myocardial demise with associated ECG changes

Stages of myocardium demise		ECG changes in area of affected myocardium	ECG trace
Ischaemia	Reduction of ventricular contraction *Reversible	Peaked (hyper acute) T waves	A
Injury	Loss of myocardial cell function *Reversible	ST elevation	B
Infarction	Death of myocardial cells *Irreversible	Q wave development, T waves inversion, R wave voltage reduction	C

away from the skin's surface during vasoconstriction, a film of sweat may appear over the patient's skin. This fluid would normally be invisible as it is evaporated by the warm blood flowing near to the skin's surface. Inhibition of insulin production can lead to an increase in blood glucose (Richards, 2005). Heart rate, respiration rate and blood pressure may increase to varying degrees as part of the sympathetic nervous response.

Occasionally patients may experience a parasympathetic nervous response (more common in inferior and posterior infarcts; see below) and experience a low heart rate and blood pressure. Relaxation of the sphincters in the bladder and anus can lead to incontinence. Increased peristalsis and tone in the gastrointestinal tract can lead to nausea and vomiting (Gray *et al.*, 2008).

In cases where cardiac output is reduced due to poor ventricular function, heart rate and respiration rate may increase to compensate for the reduction in oxygen supply to the tissues. The patient may feel breathless in the presence of pulmonary oedema (Gray *et al.*, 2008).

Chest pain is the most common presenting feature, although it must be acknowledged that 20–30% of STEMI patients will present with little or no pain. Women, older adults and people with heart failure or diabetes are commonly found in this group (Moser and Riegel, 2008). Chest pain needs to be assessed to rule out differential diagnosis (*see* Chapter 3). Pain can accurately be assessed using the PQRST mnemonic (Table 7.2). When present, the pain secondary to STEMI may be described by the patient as:

- retrosternal
- "heavy", "crushing", "squeezing", "vice-like", "throbbing" or "like a band around the chest"
- radiating to anywhere from the umbilicus to the jaw and throat but commonly the left shoulder and ulner region of the left arm
- diffuse and difficult to pinpoint
- constant, and does not differ on movement or inspiration
- not being relieved by nitroglycerin
- coming on at rest and unrelieved by rest
- lasting in excess of 20 minutes (Thygesen *et al.*, 2007).

Table 7.2 PQRST assessment of chest pain with indications for STEMI

PQRST mnemonic for chest pain assessment		Findings associated with STEMI
P	Precipitating or Palliating factors	Pain constant, can start at rest, unrelieved by rest, breathing or movement
Q	Qualitative factors	Tightness, heaviness, pressure, constriction, burning, difficult to pin point (clenched fist over central chest normally used to demonstrate – Levine's sign)
R	Region and Radiation	Retrosternal, radiating to anywhere from the lower jaw to the epigastrium but commonly ulner aspect of the arms and hands
S	Severity and associated Symptoms	Ranges from "worse pain ever" to mild pain. Measure using a numerical rating scale from 1 to 10. Associated symptoms include sweating, dyspnoea, nausea, vomiting, weakness, anxiety, pallor
T	Timing	Lasts in excess of 20 minutes

Care priorities

Assessment and diagnosis

Patients presenting with the clinical signs of STEMI need a rapid targeted assessment to confirm diagnosis (see Chapter 3 for full details). This will include the following.

Physiological assessment using the ABCDE approach

This approach outlined in Wood and Rhodes (2003) provides a systematic way of identifying immediate or potentially life-threatening abnormalities. Assessment of airway, breathing, circulation, neurological deficit (disability) and exposure will help to prioritise care and provide diagnosis (see Chapter 4). It should be noted that during assessment of circulation, blood pressure and pulse should be checked in both arms (a deficit may indicate aortic dissection) (Jowett and Thompson, 2007).

Cardiac history and physical examination

This should focus on the cardiovascular system (as detailed in Chapter 3). This may not reveal any obvious clinical signs but will help to rule out differential diagnosis. This stage of the assessment should include:

- history taking, including account of the events leading up to admission
- the identification of any risk factors for cardiac disease (see Chapter 4)
- inspection, which may reveal hyperlipidemia, peripheral vascular disease, raised jugular venous pressure (JVP) in right ventricular infarct or existing heart failure
- palpation, which may reveal apex beat displaced outwards and valve abnormalities including mitral regurgitation secondary to papillary muscle dysfunction or rupture and tricuspid regurgitation in right ventricular infarction
- auscultation, which may reveal the presence of a new murmur. The presence of a significant new murmur could suggest valvular dysfunction, such as acute mitral regurgitation or even ventricular septal rupture.

Recording of a 12-lead ECG

This should be performed immediately on arrival at hospital. ST elevation of 1mm or more in two or more adjacent limb leads and 2mm or more in two adjacent precordial (chest) leads is indicative of STEMI, as is a new conductive defect such as a new left bundle branch block (LBBB) (Conover, 2003). Posterior infarction often presents as ST depression in leads V_1 and V_2 (mirroring posterior wall ST elevation). A posterior lead ECG (utilising V_7, V_8 and V_9) may be recorded to confirm diagnosis. A patient presenting with ST elevation in the inferior limb leads will require a V_4R to identify right ventricular involvement (see below).

Blood tests

These should include the following.

- Urea and electrolytes:
  - abnormal potassium levels are associated with an increased risk of cardiac arrhythmias such as the life-threatening ventricular tachycardia and ventricular fibrillation and should be corrected as a priority in STEMI.
- Random glucose.
- Random cholesterol.
- Full blood count.
- Cardiac enzymes:
  - sensitive and specific cardiac biomarkers such as troponin (I or T) or CK-MB are recommended to aid diagnosis. These proteins leak from damaged myocytes and can be detected in the blood. Rise in their levels coupled with evidence of ischemia indicates MI. Without evidence of ischemia the rise could be secondary to an alternative cause such as myocarditis, pulmonary embolism or aortic dissection (Thygesen *et al.*, 2007)
  - blood samples for both markers should be taken on admission and 6–9 hours later. A third sample at between 12 and 24 hours is sometimes taken if previous tests are inconclusive yet suspicion of MI remains high. Serum troponin levels peak at 12 hours and thus an undetectable 12-hour level is important to exclude myocardial events. The timing of blood samples will be guided by local protocol
  - cardiac biomarkers should not be used to inform reperfusion decisions in order to prevent unnecessary delays in treatment.

Chest X-ray

Chest X-ray should be performed as routine during acute admission but should not delay treatment, unless differential diagnosis of the patient's presenting symptoms is expected. In this case chest X-ray can assist in confirming an alternative cause.

Treatment priorities

The primary aim of treatment for STEMI is to return myocardial perfusion and reduce infarct size. There has recently been a move away from thrombolysis towards primary percutaneous coronary intervention (PPCI) as the first-line treatment for AMI. This relies on local facilities and expertise, and where an acceptable PPCI service cannot be established, pre-hospital thrombolysis is recommended (DH, 2008). While reperfusion therapy is of paramount importance, other supportive treatments will help to maximise the amount of salvageable myocardium (this is explored in detail in Chapter 8 and in summary below; *see* Tables 7.3 and 7.4).

Table 7.3 Supportive pharmacology indicated in STEMI

Supportive pharmacology	Indications and current debate
Aspirin 150–325 mg oral (ESC, 2008)	Platelet aggregation inhibitor
Oxygen therapy ESC (2008) BTS (2008)	Recommends administering oxygen therapy to those who are breathless or showing signs of heart failure Recommend that oxygen should not be used to treat breathlessness but hypoxaemia: • only be given for hypoxaemic patients to maintain saturations of 94–98% or 88–92% initially for patients at risk of hypercapnic respiratory failure • be delivered via nasal specula at 2–6 l/min or simple face mask at 5–10 l/min Nurses should give oxygen as prescribed and document clearly the rate of oxygen administered and oxygen saturations achieved
Pain relief with IV morphine (AHA, 2008). Diamorphine 2.5–5.0 mg IV is given at 1 mg/min followed by 2.5 mg doses until pain is relieved (Jowett and Thompson, 2007).	Comfort of the patient and reduced workload of the myocardium • Both pain and anxiety will stimulate sympathetic nervous response resulting in peripheral vasoconstriction, increased venous return and subsequently increased myocardial workload These drugs need to be given by appropriately trained staff, clearly documented following local controlled drug policy and their effects monitored and documented to guide further treatment
Metoclopramide 5–10 mg or cyclizine 50 mg IV	Can be given with morphine to reduce the risk of nausea and vomiting (Cam, 2002)
Clopidogrel 300–600 mg loading dose followed by 75 mg daily thereafter	Patients undergoing PPCI There is conflicting guidance on whether clopidogrel should be given for STEMI patients receiving thrombolysis. The ESC (2008) recommends a loading dose of 300 mg if <75 years followed by 75 mg daily dose for all patients following STEMI for 12 months. However, NICE (2007) does not recommend the routine administration of clopidogrel and if clopidogrel is started during the acute phase it should be reviewed after four weeks. Health practitioners need to be guided by local policy

Table 7.3 *(continued)*

Supportive pharmacology	Indications and current debate
Beta blockade Commonly used beta-blockers include atenolol, bisoprolol, carvedilol, metoprolol, propranolol and sotalol	Use of routine IV beta blockade during the acute phase has been debated, but the use of oral therapy is still recommended where it is not contraindicated (e.g. heart failure, asthma or hypotension)
	IV administration is still indicated for patients who are hypertensive or tachycardic on admission (AHA, 2008; ESC, 2008) Long-term beta blockade for secondary prevention should be provided for all tolerant patients (NICE 2007).
Angiotensin-converting enzyme (ACE) inhibitor	ACE inhibitors given in the first 24h post STEMI lead to a small but significant reduction in mortality
	ACE inhibitors are recommended strongly for patients with heart failure in the early phase and/or an ejection fraction <40% • The benefits have to be weighed against the possible adverse effects of hypotension and renal failure, particularly in low-risk patients, e.g. those with a small inferior infarct (ESC, 2008)
	Long-term therapy with ace inhibitors for all STEMI patients regardless of LV function for secondary prevention has been advised by NICE (2007), but their use is not recommended as mandatory for normotensive patients without reduced LV function by ESC (2008)

Complications of STEMI

Complications post STEMI can include heart failure, ranging from mild failure to cardiogenic shock. This can be a consequence of arrhythmias or mechanical faults such as valve impairment, aneurysm, cardiac rupture or ventricular septal defect. Performing an ECG and echocardiography can help determine the cause. Other complications include pericarditis and continued ischemia. Dressler's syndrome occurs in approximately 1-5% of infarcts and results from an auto immune reaction in the first few weeks following infarction. Dressler's syndrome includes features such as malaise, pericarditis, fever, pleural effusion, anaemia and raised inflammatory markers. Treatment may have to be continued for several months and

Table 7.4 Supportive nursing investigations and care indicated in STEMI

Supportive nursing care and interventions	Indications
Immediate bed rest	Reduce physical activity and myocardial oxygen demand
Insert a wide-bore IV cannula (e.g. 14 gauge)	To prepare for the urgent administration of treatment as required
Frequent observation of vital signs including heart rate, blood pressure, respiration rate, oxygen saturations and temperature	Physiological compromise can be sudden. The frequency of measurements will depend on the stability of the patient but should generally not be left longer than 30 min each time, moving to 4-hourly once the patient is stable (Moser and Riegel, 2008)
Continuous ECG monitoring	Life-threatening rhythms such as VT, VF and asystole are common in STEMI
Serial ECGs	To detect evolving infarction
Reassurance and clear communication	To reduce anxiety and promote patient autonomy and partnership in care

includes non-steroidal anti-inflammatory agents or steroids in severe cases (Swanton, 2003).

Patients should be assessed for risk of further re-infarction, late arrhythmias or death during the acute phase. This is becoming less urgent in the advent of PPCI as coronary investigation occurs at this point.

Territories of STEMI: special considerations

The area or territory of myocardial necrosis will depend on which coronary artery is occluded. See Table 7.5 and Figure 7.3 for infarct territories in relation to ST elevation on the 12-lead ECG.

ST elevation follows the flow of coronary arteries and there is a relationship between the amount of ST elevation and the size of myocardium at risk.

Anterior STEMI

Anterior infarct has been identified as a significant independent predictor of early mortality in clinical trials (Lee et al., 1995). Left ventricular function begins to decline at the point of coronary artery occlusion even before any damage has been done to the myocardium. Continued ischaemia and damage to the myocardial cells within the left ventricle leads to further reduction in LV function. As the force of contraction diminishes the left ventricle is unable to empty efficiently into the aorta and the pressure within the ventricle

Table 7.5 Regions of STEMI and associated ECG changes

MI region	Artery occluded	Leads showing ECG changes
Anterior	LAD	V_2–V_5: anteroseptal infarction produces changes in one or more leads of V_1-V_4 (*see* Figure 7.4)
Inferior	Right (usually)	II, III, aVF "inferior leads" (*see* Figure 7.5) (Record right-sided ECG – leads V_{3R} and V_{4R} are clinically significant) (*see* Figures 7.6 and 7.7)
Posterior	Right or circumflex	Difficult to see. Posterior wall infarction causes dominant R wave (not q wave) in V_1 with ST depression (*see* Figure 7.8) Often associated with inferior MI (posterior 12-lead ECG recommended – leads V_7-V_9 are clinically significant)
Lateral	Circumflex or diagonal branch of LAD	I, aVL, $V_{5,6}$ "lateral leads"

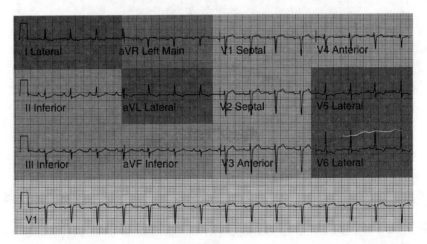

Figure 7.3 Diagrammatic representation of infarct territories in relation to the 12-lead ECG.

increases. This in turn results in a rise in pressure in the pulmonary vasculature and fluid is forced through the alveolar membrane leading to pulmonary oedema. The reduction in cardiac output that ensues often leads to powerful vasoconstriction via the sympathetic nervous system to try to maintain blood pressure to the vital centres.

Patients with STEMI (particularly anterior) can present with varying degrees of heart failure ranging from acute left ventricular failure (LVF) to cardiogenic shock (see Table 7.6).

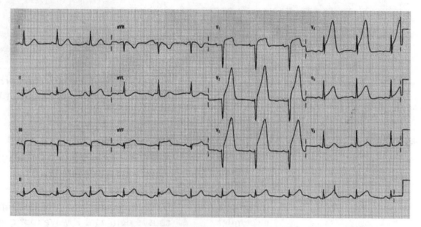

Figure 7.4 ECG demonstrating marked ST and T wave abnormalities indicative of a hyperacute STEMI of recent onset. ST elevation can be seen in V₁ through to V₅, and also in leads II, III and aVF. There is some ST depression in leads I and aVL.

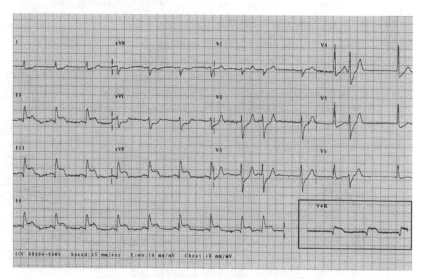

Figure 7.5 ECG showing ST segment elevation in leads II, III and aVF, which is indicative of an inferior STEMI. This patient also had a right-sided ECG recorded (see Figure 7.6), which demonstrates right ventricular involvement too.

Left ventricular failure (LVF) post STEMI

Left ventricular failure can be sudden in onset and patients may present with:

- dyspnoea with persistent pulmonary basal crepitations (rales)
- increased respirations
- low oxygen saturations

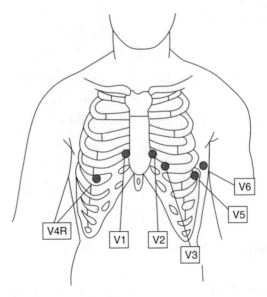

Figure 7.6 Performing a V₄R ECG.

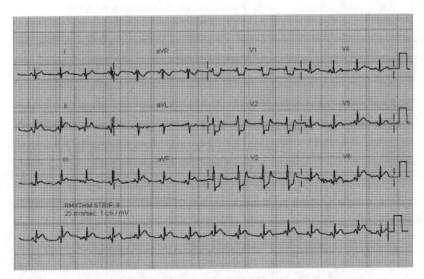

Figure 7.7 ECG showing changes indicative of a posterior STEMI. V₁ through to V₃ show the mirror image of an anteroseptal MI. There is increased R wave amplitude across these leads (a "pathologic R wave" is a mirror image of a "pathologic Q wave"). There are hyperacute ST-T wave changes, i.e. ST depression and large, inverted T waves in V₁₋₃. There is late normalisation of ST-T with symmetrical upright T waves in V₁₋₃.

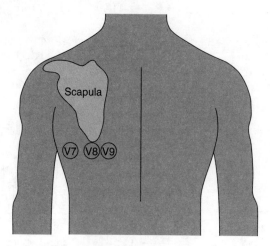

Figure 7.8 Performing a posterior lead ECG.

Table 7.6 Killip classification for heart failure post MI

Killip class	Clinical status	Mortality
1	No failure present	6%
2	Mild/moderate heart failure, some rales (crackles) present in lung fields	17%
3	Severe heart failure (frank pulmonary oedema, rales present in majority of lung fields)	38%
4	Cardiogenic shock	81%

Killip and Kimball (1967).

- cyanosis
- anxiety
- hypertension (sympathetic tone) and later hypotension as compensatory mechanisms fail
- tachycardia
- pallor and cold clammy skin
- a prominent third heart sound
- extensive necrosis may lead to cardiogenic shock, bundle branch block or heart block (Chizner, 2006; Thompson and Webster, 2004).

Patients in LVF should be assessed using the ABCDE framework (*see* Chapter 4) to prioritise needs and managed as follows.

- Sit patient up to aid breathing.
- Give oxygen as prescribed:
    - BTS (2008) recommends 2-6l/min via nasal specs or 5-10l/min via facial mask to maintain oxygen saturations of 94-98% (or 88-92% in patients with chronic obstructive pulmonary disease).

- Diuretics (loop) to reduce volume overload and the left ventricular filling pressure, e.g. 50–100 mg IV furosemide as prescribed.
- Vasodilators as prescribed to reduce afterload and improve ventricular emptying:
  - nitrates (e.g. IV GTN titrated up according to BP tolerance) are commonly used to reduce ventricular preload and improve collateral blood flow to the ventricle.
- Administer pain relief and anti-emetic as prescribed to reduce pain and anxiety and reduce myocardial oxygen demand.
- Patients will require reassurance and a calm environment.
- Beta-blockers should be withheld until patients are haemodynamically stable.
- Correct any ongoing ischaemia or arrhythmias

(Jowett and Thompson, 2007; Nolan *et al.*, 1998).

Inotropes increase myocardial contractility usually by increasing the level of calcium in the myocardial cells. Common inotropes used for LVF include dopamine and dobutamine. However, inotopes are avoided in STEMI patients in heart failure due to their stimulating effect on myocardial workload. Inotropes will increase the oxygen demand of myocardial tissue that is already depleted of oxygen. Inotropes may also trigger arrhythmias leading to further myocardial compromise.

Inferior STEMI

Patients with an inferior STEMI may present with the following.

- Hypotension and bradycardia (up to 50% of patients with inferior STEMI). The cause of these symptoms differs from the cause of hypotension found in anterior infarct. It has been found that the inferior and posterior walls of the myocardium are more prone to vagal sensory innervations (Jowett and Thompson, 2007). Vagal stimulation reduces blood pressure and heart rate even in the presence of preserved ventricular function.
- The RCA that is often occluded in inferior STEMI is usually involved in supplying the SA and AV node with oxygenated blood. An alternative cause of hypotension and bradycardia in inferior STEMI could be ischaemia of the SA and AV node. Gradual progression of heart block is not uncommon (Chizner, 2006).

As the AV node recovers over the next few hours and days following inferior infarct normal sinus rhythm usually returns.

In bradycardic patients who are symptomatic:

- withhold beta-blockers
- give atropine as prescribed

- if unsuccessful and the patient continues to be symptomatic, then a temporary pacing may be indicated (Thompson and Webster 2004).

Right ventricular STEMI

Thirty to fifty percent of patients with inferior infarction can present with varying degrees of right ventricular involvement. This is a consequence of the right ventricle being perfused by the same coronary artery as the inferior surface. In right ventricular infarction, commonly the right coronary artery (RCA), proximal to the right ventricular marginal branches, is occluded.

Patients presenting with STEMI identified in the inferior leads who become hypotensive can be mistakenly diagnosed with cardiogenic shock secondary to poor LV function. However, determining the cause of the hypotension is imperative in order to provide appropriate treatment. Patients with a right ventricular MI will usually require very different treatment than patients with poor LV function. As the function in the right ventricle is reduced, its ability to move blood into the pulmonary circulation is reduced. The build-up of pressure forces blood back into the peripheral venous system. Treatment aims to increase the stretch in the right ventricle to improve the force of contraction, thus moving the blood forwards into the pulmonary circulation.

Patients with right ventricular infarction will require:

- intravascular volume expansion in order to increase preload
    - This will use Starling's law, increasing the stretch in the right ventricle and so increasing contraction thus improving cardiac output
- Vasodilators such as opioids, nitrates, diuretics and ACE inhibitors should be avoided as they will reduce preload
- atrial fibrillation (AF), a common complication of right ventricular MI, should be promptly corrected to maximise ventricular filling from the atrium (normal atrial contraction provides 20% of ventricular end diastolic volume).

This is in stark contrast to those who are hypotensive secondary to poor LV function who usually respond better to a reduction in intravascular volume and reduced pre- and afterload (ESC, 2008).

Performing a V_4R ECG is necessary to provide diagnosis (see Figure 7.6). New ST elevation of >1mm in V_4R will identify right ventricular injury and has been said to be a predictor of short-term complications and death (Jowett and Thompson, 2007). Q waves in this lead will identify infarcted right ventricular tissue. Other clinical signs include the classical triad (Deo et al., 2005):

- raised JVP
- hypotension
- clear lung fields.

Posterior STEMI

Fifty-three percent of patients with inferior myocardial infarction will have posterior wall involvement and it is normally associated with occlusion of the right coronary artery or circumflex (Brady *et al.*, 2001). Diagnosis of posterior infarction on the ECG can be difficult as none of the 12 leads looks at the posterior surface of the heart. Usually a dominant R wave with ST depression can be seen in lead V_1 which is a reflective "mirror" image of the changes found in an anterior infarction; these are representative of changes within the posterior surface (*see* Figure 7.7). An ECG using posterior placement of electrodes is necessary to confirm diagnosis. V_7, V_8 and V_9 should be placed in the left posterior axilla line, left mid-scapula and half way between the left mid-scapula and the spine (*see* Figure 7.8).

Cardiogenic shock post STEMI

Cardiogenic shock occurs in approximately 7% of patients with STEMI. Although it can be a complication of AMI generally, it is most commonly associated with cases where the left ventricle is more than 40% damaged (Rosendorff, 2005). The result of extensive damage to the left ventricle is the insufficient supply of oxygen and nutrients to organs and tissues within the body. Without fast and effective treatment multi-organ failure will ensue. Consequently cardiogenic shock carries a high mortality rate (see Table 7.5). It is characterised by:

- persistent hypotension of <90 mm Hg systolic
- oliguria (<20 ml urine/h)
- hypoperfusion (cold extremities, mental agitation)
- cold, sweaty and cyanosed patient with rapid shallow respirations and tachycardia.

An echocardiogram will help determine the cause of the shock and guide treatment. Cardiac output will need to be restored and treatment will aim to minimise the infarct size and reduce the workload of the myocardium. Shock secondary to infarcted myocardium carries a very high mortality risk and although evidence is not conclusive, general recommendation is for patients to receive PPCI as soon as possible (SHOCK trial; Hochman *et al.*, 1999). This may require patient transfer to an interventional centre as a matter of urgency. Although mortality was not improved in cardiogenic shock patients who received thrombolysis, longer-term benefits were found in the survivors who did receive treatment (Nguyen *et al.*, 2007).

While waiting revascularisation, patients will initially need early stabilisation including:

- the correction of any electrolyte imbalance
- the correction of acid-base balance

- the prompt detection and treatment of any heart rhythm abnormality
- management of vital signs.

Treatment will include (Thompson and Webster, 2004):

- the titration of inotropes such as dobutamine and dopamine to increase cardiac contraction and improve renal perfusion. The patient will need to observed for tachycardias and arrhythmias
- diuretic therapy to reduce cardiac filling pressures, although given with caution so as not to worsen hypotension
- vasodilators such as IV GTN to reduce cardiac pre- and afterload
- fluid replacement may be required to maximise ventricular filling and reach the optimum pulmonary artery wedge pressure. However, this should be done with caution
- relief of pain and ischaemia
- control and prevention of arrhythmias
- a supportive intra-aortic balloon pump to reduce afterload and improve coronary perfusion will assist cardiac output during myocardial recovery or until reperfusion via mechanical repair can be organised
- high-flow oxygen therapy at 15 l/min (BTS, 2008).

Nurses managing this patient group will need to make frequent assessment of their patient's haemodynamic status, including fluid balance, blood pressure and, if available, pulmonary artery (PA) and PA wedge pressure (PAWP). Urinary catheterisation using an hourly measuring device is essential. Review of post STEMI medication that may worsen hypotension is required. Ideally patients should be allocated their own nurse and kept fully informed of their care at all times.

PA catheterisation

PA catheterisation may be considered to enable the assessment of PA pressure to determine the nature of the hypotension (confirming adequate left ventricular filling pressure and poor ventricular function rather than hypovolaemia) and guide treatment strategies. PAWP indicates as accurately as possible the pressure in the left ventricle at the end of diastole. The higher the pressure in the ventricle at the end of diastole the more compromised the left ventricle. Pressure indications are as follows.

- In a healthy left ventricle the end diastolic pressure should give a wedge pressure of 6-12 mm Hg.
- The point of best stretch using Starling's law is when the pressure in the left ventricle is approximately 16-18 mm Hg to aid ventricular filling.
- A PAWP of >20 mm Hg confirms cardiogenic shock.

PA catheterisation is rarely used in today's dynamic practice and requires local facilities and expertise; although this form of pressure monitoring can give a useful insight into haemodynamic status it has been suggested that it does not result in improved clinical outcomes (Moser and Riegel, 2008). Patients who have been recently thrombolysed will have added risks of haemorrhage following central vein cannulisation.

Special patient groups

Diabetes

Patients with diabetes who present with STEMI have a poorer prognosis and significantly increased mortality risk after the event than non-diabetic patients. This may be due to their reduced ability to develop collateral coronary blood supply leading to a greater reduction in LV function following an ischaemic event. Patients with diabetes often present with dyspnoea for this reason. Twenty-three percent of diabetic patients will present with STEMI without chest pain, often prolonging the time to treatment (Nguyen et al., 2007). This is a concern, considering the amount of MI patients with diabetes is already at 20% and had been said to be on the rise (Donahue et al., 2007). Alongside this, patients with or without known diabetes with blood glucose >6.7 mmol/l on admission have also been found to have higher mortality risk (Sala et al., 2002). Rapid blood sugar control on admission and thereafter for all hyperglycaemic patients with STEMI is required to reduce this risk. There has been some debate over whether control should be attained through insulin infusion in the acute phase followed by standard insulin, standard insulin from the outset or standard oral therapy (Malmberg et al., 2005) and so treatment should be guided by local protocol.

Ethnic minority groups

It has been recognised for a number of years that migrants from South Asia who reside in the UK have a higher incidence of CHD and the onset is at a younger age. Migrants from South Asia were three times more likely to have CHD below the age of 40 than the rest of the population (Balarajan, 1991). The BHF (2008) reports that male migrants from South Asia and Eastern Europe and female migrants from South Asia still have a higher death rate than the UK average. Data from 2003 show that Bangladeshi men and Pakistani women have a higher death rate than the national average by 112% and 146% respectively.

A recent study comparing the risk of MI for people from South Asia with other countries found that the mean age of AMI was 53 years (51.9 years in Bangladesh) compared with 58.8 years in other countries. The percentage of South Asian people with AMI younger than age 40 in the study was 8.9% compared with 5.6% in other countries. The study attributed this difference to a higher level of harmful risk factors and lower level of protective factors in the South Asian population, including higher levels of dyslipidemia, diabetes, anxiety and depression, and lower levels of physical activity, alcohol, and fruit and vegetable consumption (Joshi *et al.*, 2007).

Despite these differences there has been concern that once admitted to hospital with an AMI, both women and black people receive less intensive treatment than men and white people (Peterson and Yancy, 2009). Between 1994 and 2002, fewer black people than white people received reperfusion therapy in America and this difference was more marked in black women, who had the highest mortality rate (Vaccarino *et al.*, 2005). The reasons for these disparities in treatment are complex (Peterson *et al.*, 2009) and open to much debate, but it highlights the need for nurses to be sensitive to the needs of individuals from different ethnic groups. The need for good communication and education is of paramount importance in the quest for equitable care. It is also important when caring for people from different ethnic backgrounds that consideration is given to pharmacological treatment. There has been some evidence that race is a factor in the differential responses to a number of treatments, including beta-blockers, isosorbide dinitrate-hydralazine and ACE inhibitors (Peterson *et al.*, 2009). The use of ACE inhibitors, for example, has been associated with greater risk of angioedema in the black and Afro-Caribbean population (Gibbs *et al.*, 1999). Use of local pharmacology guides such as the British National Formulary will help guide treatment.

Women

The mortality rate for women with CHD is high and is the most prominent cause of death for women in the UK. CHD accounts for four times as many female deaths as cancer, with 54,491 women dying of CHD in 2001 alone (BHF, 2003). Women often present with CHD at an older age and with more co-morbidities than men, yet women may receive less intensive treatment than men with suspected MI (Vaccarino *et al.*, 2005). This could be due to the higher incidence of "atypical" presentation in women. A recent American study (Canto *et al.*, 2007) analysed 69 previous studies and found that 37% of women (versus 27% of men) were less likely to report chest pain or discomfort. Patients without typical chest pain may present with a combination of dyspnoea, fatigue, indigestion, palpitations and confusion. Others may have atypical chest pain described as not severe or prolonged, burning, sharp or positional, or focused in the arms, shoulders or neck. The atypical presentation in some women may lead to a detrimental delay in seeking help. A British study found that women were less likely than men to recognise their symptoms as requiring urgent treatment and were more difficult for health practitioners to interpret (Albarran *et al.*, 2007).

The WISE study (Lerman and Sopko, 2006) found that 50% of women presenting with suspected myocardial ischaemia who underwent investigation did not have obstructed coronary disease. However, the study recommended that physicians should not attribute evidence of ischaemia from exercise testing or biochemical markers as false-positive results. Many of these women may have microvascular ischaemia that demands intensive medical management and risk factor reduction.

Women admitted with AMI need education about signs and symptoms and risk factor reduction to improve secondary prevention. Nurses need to be sensitive to the needs of individual women and take into account cultural and ethnic diversity.

Continuing care

Once stable, the patient will require close observation over the following few days to detect any further complications. Patients should have their full lipid profile (low-density lipid, high-density lipid and very low-density lipid), renal function and glucose levels checked during this time. Nurses play a key role in educating patients about their condition and advising them about secondary prevention and returning to their normal activities. Patients who have had an uncomplicated STEMI should be mobilsed early. The first day after the event should only involve light activities, including sitting out, eating and using the commode. From the second day, gradually increased activity and walking is advised for the next few days until discharge.

Nurses should be aware that the risk of depression following MI is high, with reports that up to 65% of AMI patients suffer from symptoms of depression, including 15–22% patients suffering major depression (Post-Myocardial Infarction Depression Clinical Practice Guideline Panel, 2009). Patients should be given the opportunity to talk about their anxieties and fears and be screened for depression using a locally agreed tool prior to discharge and in the post-discharge period. Diagnosis and management of depression is important and has been linked with increase risk of morbidity and mortality in patients post STEMI.

Rehabilitation and secondary prevention

All patients should be offered cardiac rehabilitation (NICE, 2007) before discharge and a management plan should be made with the patient, taking into account their individual needs and preferences (this is covered extensively in Chapters 13 and 14).

Summary

As nurses expand their scope of practice they play an ever more important role in the management of patients who present with STEMI. This chapter has critically examined the assessment, diagnosis and priorities of care for this patient group in order to provide relief of pain and anxiety, reduce infarct size and aid speedy recovery. Nurses need an in-depth understanding of the variety of STEMI patient presentations so that they can provide prompt, evidenced-based treatments, and respond quickly and appropriately to physiological compromise. The treatment regimes discussed in this chapter embraces the recent guidance from the European Society of Cardiology, American Heart Association, NICE and British Thoracic Society.

References

Albarran J, Clarke B and Crawford J (2007) "It was not chest pain really, I can't explain it!" An exploratory study on the nature of symptoms experienced by women during their myocardial infarction. *Journal of Clinical Nursing* **16**: 1292-301.

American Heart Association (2008) 2007 Focused update of the acc/ahat 2004 guidelines for the management of patients with ST-elevation myocardial infarction. *Circulation* **117**: 296-329.

Balarajan R (1991) Ethnic differences in mortality from ischaemic heart disease and cerebrovascular disease in England and Wales. *British Medical Journal* **302**: 560-4.

Brady W, Erling B, Pollack M and Chan T (2001) Electrocardiographic manifestations: acute posterior wall myocardial infarction. *Journal of Emergency Medicine* **20**: 391-401.

British Heart Foundation (2008) Coronary Heart Disease Statistics 2008: Morbidity.

British Heart Foundation (2003) *Take Note of Your Heart: A Review of Women and Heart Disease in the UK*. London, BHF. Found at www.bhf.org.uk/heart (accessed 1 January 2008).

British Thoracic Society (2008) *Guideline for Emergency Oxygen Use in Adult Patients*. London, British Thoracic Society.

Cam A (2002) Cardiovascular disease. In: Kumar P and Clark M (eds) *Clinical Medicine* (5e). London, WB Saunders.

Canto J, Goldberg R, Hand M *et al.* (2007) Symptom presentation of women with acute coronary syndromes, myth versus reality. *Archives of Internal Medicine*. **167**(22): 2405-13.

Chizner M (2006) *Clinical Cardiology Made Ridiculously Simple*. Miami, Medmaster.

Conover M (2003) *Understanding Electrocardiography* (8e). St Louis, Mosby.

Deo R, Cannon C and Lemos J (2005) ST segment elevation myocardial infarction. In: Rosendorff C (ed.) *Essential Cardiology, Principles and Practice* (2e). New Jersey, Humana Press.

Department of Health (2008a) *Treatment of Heart Attack National Guidance: Final Report of the National Infarct Angioplasty Project (NIAP)*. London, Department of Health.

Donahue S, Stewart G, McCabe C *et al.* (2007) Diabetes and mortality following acute coronary syndromes. *Journal of the American Medical Association* **298**: 767-75.

European Society of Cardiology (2008) Management of acute myocardial infarction in patients presenting with persistent ST-segment elevation. *European Heart Journal* **29**: 2909-45.

Gibbs C, Lip G and Beevers D (1999) Angioedema due to ACE inhibitors: increased risk in patients of African origin. *British Journal of Clinical Pharmacology* **48**(6): 861-5.

Gray H, Dawkins K, Morgan J and Simpson I (2008) *Cardiology, Lecture Notes* (5e). Oxford, Blackwell Publishing

Hochman J, Sleeper L, Webb J *et al.* (1999) Early revascularization in acute myocardial infarction complicated by cardiogenic shock. SHOCK Investigators. Should we emergently revascularize occluded coronaries for cardiogenic shock. *New England Journal Medicine* **341**(9): 625-34.

Joshi P, Islam S, Pais P *et al.* (2007) Risk factors for early myocardial infarction in South Asians compared with individuals in other countries. *Journal of the American Medical Association* **297**(3): 286-94.

Jowett N and Thompson D (2007) *Comprehensive Coronary Care* (4e). London, Elsevier.

Killip T and Kimball J (1967) Treatment of myocardial infarction in a coronary care unit: two years experience with 250 patients. *American Journal of Cardiology* **20**: 457-64.

Lee K, Woodlief L, Topol E *et al.* (1995) Predictors of 30-day mortality in the era of reperfusion for acute myocardial infarction. Results from an international trial of 41,021 patients, GUSTO-1 Investigators. *Circulation* **91**: 1659-68.

Lerman A and Sopko G (2006) Women and cardiovascular heart disease: clinical implications from the women's ischemia syndrome evaluation (WISE) study. *Journal of the American College of Cardiology* **47**(3): 59S-62S.

Malmberg K, Ryden L, Wedel H *et al.* (2005) Intense metabolic control by means of insulin in patients with diabetes mellitus and acute myocardial infarction (DIGARMI 2): effects on mortality and morbidity. *European Heart Journal* **26**: 650-61.

Moser D and Riegel B (2008) *Cardiac Nursing; A Companion to Braunwald's Heart Disease*. St Louis, Saunders, Elsevier.

Myocardial Ischaemia National Audit Project (MINAP) (2008) *How the NHS Manages Heart Attacks: Seventh Public Report 2008*. London, Royal College of Physicians.

NICE (2007) *MI: Secondary prevention in Primary and Secondary Care for Patients Following a Myocardial Infarction*. London, NICE.

Nolan J, Greenwood J and Mackintosh A (1998) *Cardiac Emergencies*. Oxford, Butterworth Heinemann.

Nguyen T, Hu D, Kim M and Grines C (eds) (2007) *Management of Complex Cardiovascular Problems* (3e). Oxford, Blackwell.

Peterson E and Yancy C (2009) Eliminating racial and ethnic disparities in cardiac care. *New England Journal of Medicine* **360**(12): 1172-4.

Post-Myocardial Infarction Depression Clinical Practice Guideline Panel (2009) AAFP guideline for the detection and management of post-myocardial infarction depression. *Annals Family Medicine* **7**(1): 71-9.

Richards A (2005) The autonomic nervous system. In: Montague S, Watson R and Herbert R (ed.) *Physiology for Nursing Practice*. London, Elsevier.

Rosendorff C (ed) (2005) *Essential Cardiology, Principles and Practice* (2e). New Jersey, Humana Press.

Sala J, Masia R and Gonzalez de Molina J *et al.* (2002) Short-term mortality of myocardial infarction patients with diabetes or hyperglycaemia during admission. *Journal of Epidemiology and Community Health* **56**(9): 707-12.

Swanton R (2003) *Cardiology* (5e). Oxford, Blackwell Science.

Thompson D and Webster R (2004) *Caring for the Coronary Patient* (2e). Oxford, Butterworth.

Thygesen K, Alpert J and White H (2007) Universal definition of myocardial infarction. *Circulation* **116**: 2634-53.

Vaccarino V, Rathore S, Wenger N *et al.* (2005) Sex differences in the management of acute myocardial infarction, 1994 through 2002. *New England Journal of Medicine* **353**(7): 671-82.

Wood I and Rhodes M (eds) (2003) *Medical Assessment Units: The Initial Management of Acute Medical Patients*. London, Whurr.

Chapter 8

Therapeutic Intervention in Acute Coronary Syndromes

Jan Keenan

Introduction

As described in Chapter 4, the term "Acute Coronary Syndromes" (ACS) is applied to a spectrum of diagnoses and includes troponin-negative and troponin-positive coronary events as well as being categorised into "non-ST elevation" and "ST elevation" acute coronary syndromes (Chapters 6 and 7). The past decade has seen developments in the way terminology is used to describe each of these events, largely due to the use of cardiac troponin I (cTnI) or T (cTnT) as a marker to establish the presence or absence of myocardial damage. Therapeutic interventions are directed at increasing myocardial perfusion and reducing myocardial oxygen demand. Early diagnosis and risk stratification along with early intervention are crucial in terms of reducing the area of ischaemia and ultimately improving patient outcome. For this reason therapeutic intervention for ACS begins as soon as the patient with possible ACS is identified. The aim of this chapter is to describe the assessment, risk stratification and therapeutic interventions commonly used in the management of people with an ACS.

Learning outcomes

At the end of this chapter the reader will be able to:

- critically discuss the importance of early risk stratification within the diagnosis and management of people with ACS
- describe, using evidence-based sources, an overview of reperfusion strategies used to treat ACS in the pre-hospital context, and in secondary and tertiary care
- describe the classification of drugs used in the management of ACS and, where relevant, their effect on action potential
- discuss the key principles of safe patient transfer to theatre or from a primary or secondary care setting to a tertiary facility for intervention (discussed further in Appendix A)

Nursing the Cardiac Patient, First Edition. Edited by Melanie Humphreys.
© 2011 Blackwell Publishing Ltd. Published 2011 by Blackwell Publishing Ltd.

Pathophysiology of ACS

The pathophysiology of coronary artery disease and ACS is described elsewhere in this book (*see* Chapters 1, 4, 6 and 7). In brief, myocardial ischaemia results from an imbalance between myocardial oxygen demand and oxygen supply and can be created by one or a combination of coronary artery narrowing, coronary artery spasm and thrombotic occlusion or near occlusion of a coronary artery. In up to 90% of cases of ST elevation myocardial infarction (STEMI) (Braunwald *et al.*, 2002) occlusion or near occlusion of a coronary artery results from a thrombotic episode arising at the site of an unstable fissured plaque. Braunwald *et al.* (2002) additionally identify dynamic coronary artery obstruction, severe coronary narrowing without spasm or thrombus, arterial inflammation and secondary unstable angina as underlying pathological contributors to ACS (Green and Tagney, 2007). Thrombus in the artery is responsible for clinical changes in 35–75% of ACS without ST elevation (Braunwald *et al.*, 2002) and results in a characteristic clinical picture leading to diagnosis which, if established early enough, leads to the most effective use of time-dependent therapeutic intervention.

Early identification of ACS

Diagnosis of ACS relies on the clinical presentation of the patient, any changes in the electrocardiogram (ECG) suggestive of ischaemia and the identified release of cardiac markers, for example myoglobin (CK-MB) and/or cardiac troponin I or T. However, none of these in isolation will confirm or refute the diagnosis and it is of great importance that the information needed to make the diagnosis is established as rapidly as possible. Box 8.1 details a simple clinical history-taking format that supports the diagnosis and raises the suspicion of ischaemic cardiac chest pain based on a clear framework; in this example using the mnemonic "OLDCART".

The clinical presentation of the patient is absolutely key to early diagnosis and it is the presenting history that leads to suspicion of ACS. One of four clinical patterns may present. For example, in non-ST elevation ACS:

- rest angina of prolonged duration (>20 minutes)
- new onset severe angina
- acceleration of previously diagnosed angina
- post-infarct angina (Wenaweser and Windecker, 2008)

with 80% experiencing angina at rest, and new onset or accelerated angina in 20%. In reality, it is rare for the patient to present with abnormal clinical findings, and although a degree of heart failure may be detectable, physical examination will rarely add to the clinical history in terms of reaching a diagnosis. Physical examination will be directed to the exclusion of non-coronary causes of chest pain, such as musculoskeletal or gastric pain,

Box 8.1 The clinical history

O: Onset – The discomfort the patient experiences, whether chest pain and/or shortness of breath, may have been preceded by shorter episodes of a similar discomfort occurring at rest or on exertion. The acute event will be unrelieved by rest and may be characterised by symptoms occurring at rest or on minimal exertion. Discomfort is usually of sudden onset and crescendo in nature.

L: Location – Discomfort or pain will be in the centre or upper chest, with radiation in to the neck, throat or jaw and into the upper arms. While predominantly left arm discomfort is a feature, radiation of the discomfort into the upper back or right arm does not exclude ACS. It would be very rare for people to be able to localise discomfort, and most patients with ACS will use both hands spread over a wide area to describe their discomfort.

D: Duration – Establishing the duration of discomfort is important in terms of identifying the time at which the discomfort is at its worst. The benefits of therapeutic intervention are time dependent and the time of onset of symptoms is therefore highly relevant.

C: Characteristics – Pain will usually be described in affective terms, that is in terms of the way in which it affects the patient, such as crushing, suffocating, tightness, heaviness and dull or deep pain. People will tend to use both hands to describe their discomfort rather than a fingertip, as pain associated with ACS can rarely be localised to a specific area.

A: Associated features – ACS is usually associated with shortness of breath. Patients will also look pale as a result of the vasomotor response and feel cool and clammy to touch. Nausea and vomiting are common.

R: Relieving factors – People who are having a heart attack will not usually want to move around as this will not help the discomfort and indeed activity increases myocardial oxygen demand and therefore exacerbates the pain. There is therefore no positional element to the discomfort and it is not reproducible, nor will it be relieved, by palpation of the chest wall.

T: Treatments – It is both natural and normal behaviour to attempt self-treatment in the event of illness. People will interpret their symptoms and may have attempted the use of over-the-counter medication such as antacids or simple analgesia to relieve their discomfort. People who have access to nitrates, for example those with previously diagnosed angina, may have used sublingual tablets or spray, which may provide momentary or partial relief but will not completely relieve their discomfort.

pericarditis, pneumothorax and aortic dissection, and to look for signs of haemodynamic instability and left ventricular dysfunction (Wenaweser and Windecker, 2008)

It is important to consider the possibility of ACS at the point of presentation for people who have out-of-hospital cardiac arrest, and indeed to consider the quite significant potential for cardiac arrest induced by myocardial ischaemia in patients with ACS after reaching hospital. At whatever point the patient presents therefore, whether in primary or secondary care, by calling an ambulance or presenting at the "front door" of a health facility, it is at the point of first contact with a health professional that the presenting history must be clearly established to raise the suspicion of ACS.

On the basis of early risk scoring to predict six-month mortality, NICE (2010) recommend early therapeutic interventions that are guided by the level of risk, including initial conservative management in the lowest risk patients and ranging to more aggressive invasive strategies in those with intermediate to highest risk, or indeed those who are at lowest risk at the point of presentation who later develop clear evidence of myocardial ischaemia (see Box 4.1).

Early therapeutic intervention

In the early stages of both ST elevation- and non-ST elevation ACS both pharmacological and non-pharmacological interventions combine to reduce myocardial oxygen demand and combine with invasive strategies to improve myocardial oxygen supply.

Non-pharmacological intervention

Immediate rest reduces the physiological demand of the myocardium in terms of workload, and a wide-bore cannula (for example 14-gauge) should be inserted in anticipation of the need for urgent or emergency intravenous access. Continuous ECG monitoring should be initiated at the point of presentation, whether pre-hospital or in the hospital setting, and the frequent monitoring of blood pressure, heart rate, oxygen saturation and respiration rate is necessary, with the frequency of observation dependent on the stability of the patient. Deterioration can be sudden, and for this reason patients should, in addition to formal recording of observations, be managed in an area where constant visual assessment is possible. If the patient continues to experience symptoms suggestive of myocardial ischaemia following an initial ECG, further ECGs should be recorded at 15-minute intervals to reassess the clinical situation and identify any change that might suggest deterioration or the need for more immediate intervention, for example the development of ST depression to ST elevation, progression of T wave inversion or the extension of an area of ischaemia. Without early initial ECG changes, as the patient's condition stabilises serial ECGs should be recorded to detect changes consistent with evolving infarction, the earliest signs of which can be very subtle, and close attention should therefore be paid to detect signs such as the development of T wave inversion.

Pharmacological intervention

The earliest pharmacological intervention demonstrated to be of benefit is the administration of a single dose of aspirin for people with and without ST elevation. It reduces the relative risk of death by 15% and the risk of non-fatal myocardial infarction (MI) by 30% in both the acute phase and in secondary prevention (Theroux *et al.*, 1988). The European Society of Cardiology (2008) advocates the use of aspirin at 150–325 mg and it is usual practice in the UK for this to be administered as a 300 mg tablet, chewed by the patient until it has been completely absorbed through the oral mucosa. Oral absorption is preferable in the acute phase as it is rapid; in the clinical situation where nausea and vomiting are common it holds a significant advantage.

Aspirin at low doses inhibits the production of thromboxane in platelets, a prostaglandin responsible for platelet stimulation and aggregation and at higher doses inhibits prostacyclin, partially responsible for localised constriction in vessel walls (Grahame-Smith and Aronson, 2002). Its clear beneficial effect in both the acute setting of STEMI and in longer-term secondary prevention was demonstrated in, among others, the ISIS-2 trial (1988; cited in Baigent *et al.*, 1998). Aspirin approximately halves the risk of death or progression to infarction in unstable angina (Grahame-Smith and Aronson, 2002).

Aspirin will be given in the pre-hospital setting by a trained paramedic, or should be administered in people who are not demonstrably allergic to aspirin at the point of presentation in the community or acute hospital setting regardless of whether the patient is already taking aspirin. A nurse can administer a single dose of aspirin using a locally agreed protocol such as a patient group direction (PGD; for guidance see www.nelm.nhs.uk/en/Communities/NeLM/PGDs/) or under prescription and it will continue indefinitely at low dose (for example 75 mg/day).

Pain control

The patient with severe cardiac pain is both distressed and in danger. Pain is associated with a physiological response mediated by the sympathetic nervous system that increases blood pressure and heart rate, and therefore myocardial oxygen demand. Increased pain can therefore result from its physiological response and exacerbates the severity of the situation. Opiates such as diamorphine (2.5–5 mg) or morphine (1–10 mg), given slowly intravenously and titrated according to response, relieve both pain and distress, and reduce sympathetic nervous system activity. Opiates dilate peripheral arterioles and venules, therefore reducing both preload and afterload, and reduce cardiac failure. Their potent anxiolytic effect is additionally beneficial in the acute phase. However, because of their physiological effects they should be used with a degree of caution, particularly in elderly people who may be very sensitive to these effects, and in patients with chronic lung disease, as they depress the respiratory centre (Grahame-Smith and Aronson, 2002). In addition, opiates can cause hypotension, nausea and vomiting. The latter are common in patients with ACS and it is therefore common practice to use anti-emetics alongside opiates to mitigate against this effect; meto-clopramide tends to be the drug of choice as it has fewer cardiovascular effects.

Oxygen

The use of oxygen therapy in ACS was at one time advocated for all patients as it was believed that increasing oxygen concentration of circulating blood improved myocardial oxygen supply (see for example the National Service Framework for CHD; DH, 2000). More recently the practice of routine oxygen administration has been challenged and the ESC (2008) guideline recommends administration of oxygen only to patients who are breathless or who are showing signs of heart failure. However, the British Thoracic Society (BTS, 2008) recommends that oxygen should not be administered to breathless patients but only to those with hypoxia in order to maintain oxygen saturations at 94–98%, or 88–92% initially for those at risk of hypercapnic respiratory failure, and delivered via nasal specula at 2–6 l/min or simple face mask at 5–10 l/min. Mayor (2010) argues that the rationale for the routine administration of oxygen for patients with MI is based on a belief that it improves oxygenation of ischaemic myocardium and therefore reduces cardiac pain and infarct size, but there is insufficient evidence to determine whether oxygen has an effect on these outcomes and in due course this may be the subject of a Cochrane systematic review. Oxygen is a drug, and while it can be administered under national protocols in the pre-hospital context (JRCALC, 2006), in the hospital context it must be prescribed and documented at the rates administered alongside the oxygen saturations achieved.

Therapeutic intervention for STE-ACS and NSTE-ACS

Following initial assessment and emergency management, the pathway for patients with ST elevation or non-ST elevation begins to diverge. The mainstay of therapy for NSTE-ACS is early identification of people at high risk, along with early pharmacological therapy and it is therefore appropriate at this point to differentiate between treatment pathways.

NSTE-ACS

The primary goal of therapy in people with NSTE-ACS is restoration of blood flow and resolution of ischaemia, and this is described well by

Wenaweser and Windecker (2008), who refer to "four pillars of acute treatment" as:

- antiplatelet agents
- anticoagulants
- anti-ischaemic therapy
- coronary revascularisation.

It is important to consider the potential benefits of antiplatelet and anticoagulant therapy in all patients with ACS, alongside what has been demonstrated to be a substantial bleeding risk in people at high risk in particular, such as those with renal failure or older people. Consideration therefore needs to be given to the use of these agents and this is guided by a cardiologist.

Angiography and revascularisation

Angiography is pivotal to determining revascularisation strategy (discussed further in Chapters 7 and 9). Revascularisation is performed to relieve angina and ongoing myocardial ischaemia and to prevent progression to STEMI or death (ESC, 2007).

Primary percutaneous coronary intervention

Primary percutaneous coronary intervention (pPCI) began in some centres in the UK in 2002 and involves both extraction of thrombus and reopening of the affected artery with intra-coronary stenting. pPCI results in more reliable opening of the coronary artery with a lower risk of stroke and early re-occlusion (see Figures 8.1, 8.2 and 8.3 for schematic representation of the process). It reduces mortality and improves long-term outcome and for this reason the NIAP report (DH, 2008) recommended transfer of STEMI patients to "heart attack" centres where there is a 24-hour-a-day, seven-day-a-week service offering pPCI and with experienced operators. There is evidence of a correlation between improved outcome and the number of procedures undertaken in a centre that supports the development of "heart attack" centres, and policy is generally driven towards the development of experience in high-volume tertiary centres (DH, 2008). pPCI should be performed if the patient presents within 12 hours of symptom onset, or later only if there is evidence of ongoing ischaemia (ESC, 2008).

However, the logistical difficulties of setting up a pPCI service mean that roll-out of pPCI at a national level is gradual, and while significant numbers of patients are now treated with pPCI, the Department of Health (2008) acknowledged that roll-out of a national service in the UK would take time, with full implementation anticipated by 2011, and while implementation in some areas outside the UK is complete, in other areas access to pPCI continues to develop at a lesser rate.

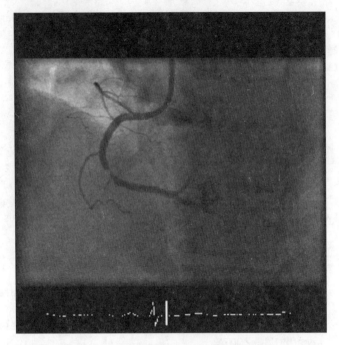

Figure 8.1 Disease of the right coronary artery (RCA).

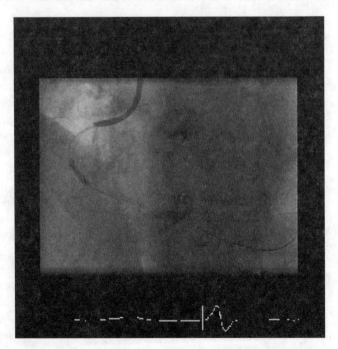

Figure 8.2 Right coronary artery disease with wire in position within the artery.

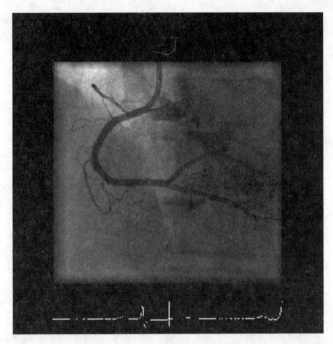

Figure 8.3 Right coronary artery PCI with stent in situ within the vessel.

Without question, the time taken to treatment for STEMI greatly influences outcome and with the advent of pPCI this is equally relevant. The time measure "call to balloon" (CTB) is a measure of likely treatment efficacy, with the greater mortality benefits seen with low CTB times at 30 days, one year and 18 months following intervention. For this reason CTB times are monitored at a national level in the UK with a recommended CTB time of no more than 120 minutes considered acceptable. Close collaboration is required between acute services, treatment centres and ambulance services to develop pathways that support immediate patient transfer, often across county or health authority boundaries, to heart attack centres for timely treatment, and for this reason the skill of the ambulance crew is paramount in identifying the patient with STEMI and transferring them directly to a heart attack centre. It does not help the patient to delay transfer by calling at a centre that cannot offer pPCI facilities in order to confirm the diagnosis, and while there can be understandable nervousness about patient stability en route, it should be noted that data supporting the benefits of pPCI came from studies that included people who were sick or unstable during transfer.

pPCI has dramatically changed the role of the coronary care unit (CCU) nurse and if the patient is admitted to a CCU in advance of pPCI, the focus of the nurse is on maintaining patient safety, nursing measures to reduce myocardial oxygen demand and increase myocardial oxygen supply, maintenance of adequate pain relief and management of early arrhythmias (see Chapter 10), along with preparation of the patient for intervention, including consent. A high loading dose (600mg) of clopidogrel may have been given pre-hospital, but if not, the nurse should administer this without delay, and again this single loading dose can be given either with a prescription or using a PGD. Similarly, according to local protocol prasugrel may be used as an alternative with a loading dose of 60mg (see above).

As pPCI services develop, so does the means by which patients are delivered to heart attack centres for intervention, including direct ambulance transfer to angiography facilities in tertiary centres to expedite treatment, and the patient may not be admitted to a CCU until after the procedure (see Appendix A for more details on safe patient transfer). Priorities in this case are initial rest and monitoring for complications of the procedure, including bleeding at the arterial access site, early stent thrombosis manifest as further chest pain with ST elevation, and the risk of early arrhythmias (see Chapter 10). Complications following the initial treatment phase remain and are directly related to the location and extent of myocardial damage. For this reason an echocardiogram to assess the extent of damage to the myocardium is invaluable, and in addition it facilitates the detection of other potential complications, such as thrombus in the left ventricle.

The majority of patients recover rapidly following pPCI and need careful management and early assessment by a cardiac rehabilitation specialist to establish a plan for early, medium- and long-term recovery. Medical therapy will include pharmacological secondary prevention, but because patients recover following pPCI there is a significant reduction in hospital stay compared with treatment with thrombolysis.

Thrombolysis

Thrombolytic therapy reduces mortality from MI, certainly up to 12 hours and possibly longer from the onset of symptoms (Grahame-Smith and Aronson, 2002). Streptokinase, alteplase, anistreplase and urokinase are all activators of plasminogen and thus cause fibrinolysis; they are summarised in Table 8.1.

Administration of thrombolysis

Thrombolytic therapies, as described above, can be administered in the pre-hospital setting or when the patient arrives in hospital. In the setting of ACS, thrombolysis is indicated only for patients presenting with ECG criteria suggesting STEMI along with a clinical presentation consistent with acute MI. Thrombolytics increase the risk of bleeding and have also been demonstrated to increase the risk of stroke. While this risk is outweighed by the benefits of improved survival following STEMI, some patients remain unsuitable for thrombolysis, for instance because they are at higher risk of bleeding (DH, 2008).

Whoever initiates thrombolytic therapy must establish whether there is any contra-indication or caution to its administration (see Box 8.2) before initiating treatment. If a thrombolytic has not been administered by a paramedic, in many areas of the UK nurses are able to administer thrombolysis

Table 8.1 Thrombolytic therapies in current UK use

Thrombolytic	Administration	Indications	Potential side effects/drawbacks	Benefits	Trial evidence
Streptokinase	1.5 million units administered by intravenous injection over one hour	STEMI, up to 12 h following the onset of symptoms	Hypotension, allergic reaction including anaphylaxis, haemorrhage	Reduced mortality compared with placebo	GISSI (1986); ISIS-2 (1988)
Alteplase (tPA)	Accelerated infusion of 100 mg over 3 h; 10% dose as a bolus over 1–2 min followed by 50% as an infusion over 1h; subsequent 40% as an infusion over 2 h (maximum 1.5 mg/kg dose in people weighing <65 kg)	Up to 12 h following symptom onset – arguably with benefit up to 24 hours where there is persistent ST elevation	Haemorrhagic and stroke risk in older people compared with streptokinase	Tolerated well in comparison with streptokinase; reduced mortality	FTT Collaborative Group (1994)
Reteplase (RPA)	Two IV bolus injections of 10 units, 30 min apart	Up to 12 h following symptom onset	Haemorrhagic risk as above; exact 30 min between bolus doses may be difficult to achieve with patient transfer	Tolerated well; ease of administration pre-hospital	INJECT study (Schröder et al., 1995)
Tenecteplase (TNK)	Single intravenous bolus over 10 s; 30–50 mg according to body weight	Up to 6 h following symptom onset	Haemorrhagic risk; difficulty in establishing weight of patient, with too high a dose markedly increasing bleeding risk	Tolerated well; ease of administration pre-hospital and in emergency setting	ASSENT-2 study (Van de Werf et al., 1999)

> ## Box 8.2   Contraindications to thrombolysis
>
> - Recent (<6 weeks): major trauma, surgery, dental extraction, menorrhagia, post partum
> - Prolonged (>20 min) CPR
> - Cerebrovascular accident within 6 months, or *any* haemorrhagic CVA or CVA of unknown aetiology
> - Coma
> - Bleeding diathesis
> - Patients taking warfarin
> - Severe liver disease
> - Severe hypertension (BP > 180/100 despite treatment)
> - Recent peptic ulcer symptoms
> - Acute pancreatitis
> - Oesophageal varices
> - Pulmonary disease with cavitation
> - Pregnancy
> - Laser therapy for retinopathy in the last week
> - Infective endocarditis
> - Pericarditis
> - History suggestive of aortic dissection
> - Known aortic aneurysm
> - Patients who have had more than 12 h of chest pain

either following a prescription or using a PGD, which allows a nurse to supply and administer a single dose of medication without a prescription under specific circumstances (Humphreys and Smallwood, 2004). In addition, the advent of non-medical prescribing has in some areas facilitated better access to timely treatment without the need for extensive protocols in this group of patients, and without need for early attendance by medical staff.

The dose and preparation of thrombolytic agents is dealt with in Table 8.1. All patients receiving thrombolysis should be managed in a high-visibility area such as a CCU, with nurses experienced in the management of sick patients. Blood pressure, heart rate and oxygen saturations should be monitored continuously and recorded every 15 minutes during the administration of infused agents. A loading dose of clopidogrel 300 mg has been demonstrated to be of benefit and in patients managed for STEMI without coronary intervention should be continued for one month. There should also be continuous assessment of pain control and opiate analgesia may need to be administered frequently to minimise discomfort, along with an anti-emetic if needed. The health professional should be alert to the potential for bleeding and if the patient's conscious level deteriorates inconsistent with the use of opiate analgesia, a member of the senior medical team should be alerted to the possibility of stroke.

Effectiveness of thrombolysis

The efficacy of thrombolytic therapy can be established relatively early following administration and is related to clinical signs suggestive of recanalisation of the affected artery. Signs of reperfusion include normalisation of the ST segment on the ECG or the development of T wave inversion, and for this reason an ECG should be recorded 60–90 minutes following the commencement of the thrombolytic. Less than 50% resolution of ST elevation suggests failure of thrombolysis, and in these circumstances medical teams should be alerted to the possibility of the need for further intervention. Accelerated idioventricular rhythm and an increase in ventricular ectopic activity have been associated with reperfusion (Doevendans et al., 1995), and the same study reported relief of chest pain after 60 minutes by 96% of patients with recanalisation of the artery following thrombolysis.

An ECG should be recorded whenever the patient has a change in their clinical condition, for example a period of idioventricular rhythm or if chest pain resolves or indeed accelerates. Despite thrombolysis, the affected coronary artery can re-occlude and further ECG changes develop, signalling the potential need for further intervention.

Drawbacks of thrombolysis

As suggested above, not all patients are suitable for thrombolysis, for instance because they have a high risk of bleeding. However, in approximately 20–30% of those who are suitable the affected artery fails to re-open following treatment (DH, 2008). Early administration of thrombolysis clearly results in a better outcome for patients, but its limitations led to the development of more mechanical means to re-open coronary arteries during the acute event, remove thrombus and insert a coronary stent, and indeed the development of pPCI.

Facilitated percutaneous coronary intervention

An alternative approach to thrombolysis or pPCI has been speculated to offer early treatment benefits for people with STEMI who cannot be provided with pPCI in a short time period. The term "facilitated PCI" has been used to refer to multiple strategies of pharmacotherapy administered before immediate PCI, including full-dose or half-dose fibrinolytic agent or GP IIb/IIIa inhibitor, as well as combinations of these two agents. Given the geographical challenges placed on services in terms of transfer times for pPCI, this has been of worthy consideration. However, the ASSENT-4 trial studying the use of full-dose tenecteplase followed by PCI versus PCI alone was stopped early due to a clearly demonstrated raised in-hospital mortality at 30 days (6% versus 3%), which was largely attributable to higher rates of stroke (Kiernan et al., 2007). Facilitated PCI recipients also had significantly higher rates of death, heart failure or shock within 90 days, as well as much higher rates of haemorrhagic stroke, re-infarction and repeat target vessel revascularization (ASSENT-4, 2006).

Subsequent meta-analyses of randomised controlled trials comparing facilitated PCI with PCI alone supported these findings, and therefore facilitated PCI is not considered a safe or effective alternative to pPCI or thrombolysis for people in geographically challenged areas.

Summary

The management of ACS is developing at a pace. Therapeutic intervention begins with identifying the patient with possible ACS and establishing the extent of risk. Pharmacological strategies for management of ACS include the use of effective antithrombotic and anticoagulant agents, followed by mechanical reperfusion for all but the lowest-risk patients. Advances in pharmacology and in revascularisation technology continue for the benefit of patients, and in particular in terms of improving long-term morbidity and mortality. The more recent development of primary PCI offers the benefit of early revascularisation and significantly improved outcomes in patients with STEMI, and can benefit a far wider group of people than thrombolysis. It represents a quantum step forward in our ability to manage people with life-threatening disease.

References

ASSENT-4 PCI Investigators (2006) Assessment of the safety and efficacy of a new treatment strategy with percutaneous coronary intervention. Primary versus tenecteplase-facilitated percutaneous coronary intervention in patients with ST-segment elevation acute myocardial infarction (ASSENT-4 PCI): randomised trial. Lancet **18**(367): 569–78.

Assessment of the Safety and Efficacy of a New Thrombolytic (ASSENT-2) Investigators, Van de Werf F, Adjey J, Ardissino D et al. (1999) Single bolus tenecteplase compared with front-loaded alteplase in acute myocardial infarction: the ASSENT-2 double-blind randomised trial. Lancet **354**(9180): 716–22.

Baigent C, Collins R, Appleby P, Parish S, Sleight P and Peto R (1998) ISIS-2: 10 year survival among patients with suspected acute myocardial infarction in randomised comparison of intravenous streptokinase, oral aspirin, both, or neither. The ISIS-2 (Second International Study of Infarct Survival) Collaborative Group. British Medical Journal **2**(316): 1337–43.

Braunwald E, Antman E, Beasley J et al. (2002) American College of Cardiology/American Heart Association Guideline for the update management of patients with unstable angina and NSTEMI: a report from the American College of Cardiology/American Heart Association Task Force on Practice Guidelines. www.acc.org/qualityandscience/clinical/guidelines/unstable/update_index.htm (accessed 11 June 2010).

British Thoracic Society (BTS) (2008) Guideline for Emergency Oxygen Use in Adult Patients. London, British Thoracic Society.

Department of Health (DH) (2008) *Treatment of Heart Attack National Guidance; Final Report of the National Infarct Angioplasty Project (NIAP).* London, Department of Health and the British Cardiovascular Society.

Department of Health (DH) (2000) *National Service Framework for Coronary Heart Disease.* London, Department of Health.

Doevendans P, Gorgeis A, van der Zee R, Partouns J, Bar F and Wellens H (1995) Electrocardiographic diagnosis of reperfusion during thrombolytic therapy in acute myocardial infarction. *American Journal of Cardiology* **75**(17): 1211-13.

European Society of Cardiology (ESC) (2008) Management of acute myocardial infarction in patients presenting with persistent ST elevation. *European Heart Journal* **29**: 2909-45.

European Society of Cardiology (ESC) (2007) Guideline for the diagnosis and treatment of non-ST segment elevation acute coronary syndromes. *European Heart Journal* **28**: 1598-660.

Fibrinolytic Therapy Trialists Collaborative Group (1994) Indications for fibrinolytic therapy in suspected acute myocardial infarction: collaborative overview of early mortality and major morbidity. Results from all RCTs of more than 1000 patients. *Lancet* **343**: 311-22.

Grahame-Smith D and Aronson J (2002) *Clinical Pharmacology and Drug Therapy* (3e). Oxford, Oxford University Press.

Green S and Tagney J (2007) Chest pain due to an acute coronary syndrome, pp. 71-94. In: Albarran J and Tagney J (eds) (2007) *Chest Pain: Advanced Assessment and Management Skills.* Oxford, Blackwell.

Gruppo Italiano per lo Studio della Streptochinasi nell'Infarto Miocardico (GISSI) (1986) Effectiveness of intravenous thrombolytic treatment in acute myocardial infarction. *Lancet* **8478**: 397-402.

Humphreys M and Smallwood A (2004) An exploration of the ethical dimensions pertinent to gaining consent for thrombolysis. *Nursing in Critical Care* **9**(6): 264-70.

Joint Royal Colleges Ambulance Liaison Committee (JRCALC) (2006) UK Ambulance Service Clinical Practice Guidelines www2.warwick.ac.uk/fac/med/research/hsri/emergencycare/prehospitalcare/jrcalcstakeholderwebsite/guidelines (accessed 18 June 2010).

Kiernan T, Ting H and Gersh B (2007) Facilitated percutaneous coronary intervention: current concepts, promises, and pitfalls. *European Heart Journal* **28**(13): 1543-5.

Mayor S (2010) Giving oxygen in acute myocardial infarction may raise death risk, Cochrane review concludes. *British Medical Journal* **340**: c3227 http://bmj.com/cgi/content/full/340/jun16_1/c3227 (accessed 21 June 2010).

NICE (2010) *Unstable Angina and NSTEMI* (NICE clinical guideline 94). London, National Institute for Health and Clinical Excellence.

Schröder R, Wegscheider K, Schröder K, Dissmann R, Meyer-Sabellek W for the INJECT trial group (1995) Extent of early ST segment elevation resolution: a strong predicator of outcome in patients with acute myocardial infarction and a sensitive measure to compare thrombolytic regimens: a substudy of the International Joint Efficacy Comparison of Thrombolytics (INJECT) trial. *Journal of the American College of Cardiology* **26**(7): 1657-64.

Theroux P, Ouimet H, McCans J et al. (1988) Aspirin heparin or both to treat acute unstable angina. *New England Journal of Medicine* **319**: 1105-11.

Wenaweser P and Windecker S (2008) Acute coronary syndromes. Management and secondary prevention. *Herz* **33**: 25-37.

Chapter 9
Cardiothoracic Care

Debbie Danitsch

Introduction

Currently, approximately 600,000 coronary artery bypass grafts (CABG) operations are performed worldwide every year. Although CABG has been performed on older and sicker patients since the inception of drug-eluting stents and the publication of the National Service Framework for the older person (Abu-Omar and Taggart, 2009; DH, 2001), mortality has remained at 2%. The main drawback following CABG is vein graft failure leading to angina, myocardial infarction and death; however, the widespread use of statins and anti-platelet drugs may increase graft longevity (Mangano, 2002).

Although there are a number of emergency procedures performed for thoracic aortic dissection and bacterial endocarditis, the most common operations performed routinely are coronary artery grafts and repair or replacement of heart valves. Transplantation is also carried out at some centres but it is beyond the scope of this chapter to cover the care of patients having emergency and transplantation surgery, and only the care of patients having routine cardiac surgery will be covered.

Learning outcomes

At the end of this chapter the reader will be able to:

- discuss the management of patients undergoing coronary artery grafting
- discuss the differing conduits used for grafting
- describe the process of open heart surgery and discuss the complications that may occur and the treatment of these complications
- understand and recognise when a patient is ready to "fast track"
- identify the needs of the patient before discharge.

Nursing the Cardiac Patient, First Edition. Edited by Melanie Humphreys.
© 2011 Blackwell Publishing Ltd. Published 2011 by Blackwell Publishing Ltd.

Preparation for surgery

Information should be given to patients before surgery as part of the process of informed consent. Providing full information to patients means ensuring that they not only understand consequences of the treatment options but also have a clear understanding of the impact of potential complications. The use of open questions can check understanding as the consultation progresses, and the verbal process can be supplemented with written information, diagrams and even audiovisual presentations. Written information plays a valuable part in reflection and patients and their relatives need to be given sufficient time to reflect in order to make valid informed consent. In addition, patients expect the person taking consent to be familiar with the procedure and to be able to answer all their questions. Ideally, this should be someone who performs the procedure regularly (www.library.nhs.uk/theatres/viewResource.aspx?resid=259250&code=60aa7050a268a407c3333b03437d2799).

Consent should be an ongoing process that begins when the patient is seen in the outpatient clinic by the surgeon. The procedure should be explained again at preadmission and informed written consent sought. If consent is delegated to another practitioner who is not the operating surgeon they should have received education and had their competency assessed by the surgeon who performs the operation. This should be updated on a yearly basis. The benefits and risks of the surgery should be explained.

Patients need to be prepared because it is important that they understand the risks associated with their surgery and are quoted figures. These figures will vary depending on the patient's individual circumstances, but all patients are at risk of:

- death
- serious arrhythmias
- embolic episodes such as stroke, pulmonary embolus or deep vein thrombosis
- chest infections and infections in wounds, including mediastinitis, which can be fatal
- haemorrhage
- renal failure and respiratory (Pedro *et al.*, 2009).

EuroSCORE

Two risk calculators often used are the simple additive EuroSCORE and the full logistic EuroSCORE. The simple additive EuroSCORE model is now well established and has been validated in many patient populations across the world. It is easy to use, even at the bedside. It is valuable in quality control in cardiac surgery and gives a useful estimate of risk in individual patients. However, particularly in very high-risk patients, the simple additive model may sometimes underestimate the risk when certain combinations of risk factors co-exist. The full logistic version of EuroSCORE produces more accurate risk prediction for a particular high-risk patient. Its main disadvantage is that the risk has to be calculated in quite a complex way – not by mental arithmetic or "on the back of an envelope" (www.mpoullis.com/euro.htm).

Pre admission clinics

In preadmission clinics patients are assessed and clerked, and a recording of the patient's history and presenting medical condition is documented. It is good practice to complete and record scores of pressure areas, nutritional status and falls risk in the preoperative period.

- The patient should be assessed for any signs of infection, including temperature recording and a white cell count.
- All routine bloods should be taken to check for any abnormalities including urea and creatinine and the patient should be cross-matched for four units of blood, in cases of redo surgery six units may be requested by some surgeons. If the patient does not want to receive blood they should be offered the opportunity to donate their own blood if their clinical condition allows and they have stable angina. This should be done 3–4 weeks before the planned surgery. If this is not possible patients should be informed of the extra risks associated with not receiving blood in the event of them haemorrhaging. The alternative fluids that can be used should also be discussed with the patient.
- A chest X-ray and electrocardiogram (ECG) should also be performed and reviewed prior to surgery to detect any changes in the patient's condition since they were last seen by the surgeon in clinic. These results provide practitioners with a baseline for managing the patient postoperatively. If the patient has a chronic or acute chest condition a routine blood gas will provide a useful guide to ventilation postoperatively.
- The patient's body surface area (BSA) needs to be calculated preoperatively, as the BSA gives a better indication of the metabolic mass than body weight alone because it is less affected by abnormal adipose mass. There are many formulas available to do this but probably the most commonly used is the Mosteller formula (Mosteller, 1987). This formula is:

$$\text{BSA (m}^2) = \text{the square root of } \frac{\text{weight (kg)} \times \text{height (cm)}}{3600}.$$

There are readily available tools in cardiothoracic units that can be used to automatically calculate this value, but the patient's height and weight need to be recorded to enable this. The normal values are $1.9\,\text{m}^2$ for men and $1.6\,\text{m}^2$ for women. These values are used for drug dose calculations and to calculate the amount of intravenous fluids required by the patient. Renal function and cardiac output measurements can also be calculated with this information.

- Echocardiographic assessment prior to valve surgery is crucial for clinical decision making, timing of surgery, planning the appropriate surgical therapy and predicting the patient's outcome (Germing and Mügge, 2009).
- Anti-platelet drugs should be stopped 5-9 days prior to surgery to reduce the risk of bleeding complications, unless specifically contraindicated (Cahill *et al.*, 2005).
- Patients should be encouraged to discuss any particular worries they have in an effort to allay their fears and a visit to the intensive care unit should be undertaken so they view the environment and machinery before they are admitted.

The operation

Traditionally, cardiac surgery is performed using a median sternotomy of 6-8 inches in length, allowing the surgeon to access the heart and put the patient on to a cardiopulmonary bypass machine. This machine bypasses the lungs and heart to enable the heart to be operated on while it is still and bloodless, and the lungs to be deflated to maximise visualisation of the operative site; it allows temporary disruption to the circulatory system without causing global ischaemia (Margerson and Riley, 2003). An alternative to traditional CABG is off-pump or beating-heart surgery, where surgeons do not use the heart-lung machine. The procedure is also called OPCAB (off-pump coronary artery bypass). The surgeons sew the bypasses onto the heart while it continues to beat. High-risk patients with additional diseases such as lung disease, kidney failure or peripheral vascular disease may benefit from this technique.

- Cardioplegia is given to arrest the heart while in theatre; *cardio* means the heart, and *plegia* means paralysis. To achieve this, deoxygenated blood entering the heart through the superior and inferior vena cavae are diverted using venous canulae to the cardiopulmonary bypass machine. This pump takes over the function of the lung by oxygenating the blood and removing carbon dioxide using an oxygenator in the circuit. After oxygenation, filtration and removal of carbon dioxide, the blood is pumped back into the body, usually through the aorta, although the femoral artery and the right axillary artery can be used.
- The heart is then isolated from the rest of the body by a cross-clamp on the aorta and cold cardioplegia is introduced into the heart through the aortic root. The blood supply to the heart arises from the aortic root through the coronary arteries. The cold fluid (usually at 4°C) ensures that the heart cools down to an approximate temperature of around 15-20°C. This is further augmented by the cardioplegia component, which is high in potassium and magnesium. The potassium helps by arresting the heart in diastole, thus ensuring that the heart does not use up the valuable

energy stores (adenosine triphosphate). Blood can be added to this solution, particularly for long procedures requiring more than half an hour of cross-clamp time. Blood acts a buffer and also supplies nutrients to the heart during ischaemia.

- During bypass conduits are used to bypass the diseased arteries enabling a superior flow to the myocardium. Conduits used are the long saphenous veins and internal mammary arteries; sometimes radial arteries are used but this is rarer. The gastro-epiploic artery has been used, but because this artery is in the abdomen it lengthens the operative time and is currently used less often than other conduits.

- Hypothermia is defined as a core temperature below 36.8°C. While hypothermia can be a consequence of many types of surgery because of the inhibition of central thermoregulation and exposure to cold operating rooms, in cardiac surgery hypothermia is induced while the patient is on the bypass machine. The rationale for the use of hypothermia is based on its capacity to reversibly reduce metabolic activity in all cells and subcellular organelles, such as the mitochondria and the nucleus of the cell, further limiting the rate of consumption of intracellular high-energy phosphate stores and limiting ischaemic injury. This results in slower metabolism and reduced cardiac demands. As well as the positive effects, hypothermia also has some negative effects, two of the most important being the delirious influence on platelet function and the increase in citrate toxicity with a reduction in serum ionised calcium. These effects can result in coagulopathies, making the patient more susceptible to bleeding in the postoperative period, and dysrhythmias with depression of myocardial contractility (Lewis *et al.*, 2002; Ning *et al.*, 1998; Tonz *et al.*, 1995).

- Advances in technology have now made it possible to perform beating heart surgery where the patient does not have to be put on a bypass machine. There are obvious benefits to this as the risks of morbidity and mortality are greatly reduced. Minimally invasive direct CABG (MIDCABG) is useful when there is one vessel disease, for example a left anterior descending artery blockage where the left internal mammary artery can be used. There have also been advances in robotically assisted surgery for MIDCABG.

- A transcatheter aortic valve implantation (TAVI) has recently been introduced for use in patients who are considered by the multidisciplinary team to be too high a risk for valve surgery. This is performed on a beating heart and avoids the need for sternotomy. It can be performed via transfemoral, subclavian or transapical approaches. Recommendations by the British Cardiovascular Society and the Society for Cardiothoracic Surgery suggest that at least 50 cases per year are performed for the procedure to be optimal (www.scts.org/documents/PDF/BCISTAVIDec2008.pdf).

Postoperative care

The main aim in the first 24 hours following cardiac surgery is haemodynamic stabilisation and minimising myocardial ischaemia (Myles *et al.*, 1997).

Careful, continuous monitoring of the patient should be undertaken with one registered nurse caring for the patient. The patient's care will be discussed using a systems approach to ensure all elements are covered.

On their return to the ward, the nurse should receive a thorough report about the patient's progress in theatre from the anaesthetist and be informed of any problems that were encountered during the operation. When the patient is stabilised, routine bloods should be checked, including an activated partial thromboplastin time (APPT) and an international normalised ratio (INR). Routine taking of chest X-rays and ECGs can no longer be justified postoperatively when there is no clinical sign of disease, but a chest X-ray following drain removal to identity pneumothorax and one ECG postoperatively should be recorded.

Respiratory

The patient should be attached to a ventilator. The mode of ventilation (pressure or volume) is less important than the achievement of optimum ventilation with appropriate tidal volumes.

- In patients with no pre-existing lung disease, volumes of 10–12 ml/kg should be achieved with a rate of 12 breaths per minute. In patients with pre-existing lung disease the tidal volume achieved should be smaller, about 8–10 ml/kg.
- Airway pressures should not exceed 45 cm H_2O in order to prevent barotrauma.
- When using volume controlled ventilation positive end expiratory pressure (PEEP) should be added at 5 cm H_2O to oppose the passive emptying of the lungs. This works by increasing the alveolar pressure and volume, which facilitates splintage of the airways. PEEP can also be used up to 10 cm H_2O to increase the airway pressure when patients are bleeding.
- After initialising ventilation, auscultation of the chest should be performed to check for bilateral air entry and ensure there is no pneumothorax or that the endotracheal tube has not slipped into the right main bronchus during the transfer from theatre.
- Arterial blood gases (ABG) should be monitored regularly to ensure ventilation is adequate and to highlight when changes are needed to optimise ventilation. Table 9.1 provides a quick reference guide, more information can be found in Coggon (2008).

After a period of stability the decision to wean and wake the patient should be made. The patient should be haemodynamically stable, bleeding should be minimal (less than 50 ml/hour for two consecutive hours), temperature should be reaching normal and oxygenation should be optimum (PO_2 greater than 10 kilopascals, kPa).

- After cardiac surgery it is common for patients to develop microatelectasis due to the fact that the lungs are collapsed during surgery and the

Table 9.1 Changes found in arterial blood gases in patients with respiratory and metabolic conditions

	pH	PaCO$_2$	HCO$_3$
Respiratory acidosis	↓	↑	Normal
Respiratory alkalosis	↑	↓	Normal
Metabolic acidosis	↓	Normal	↓
Metabolic alkalosis	↑	Normal	↑

anaesthetic gases used decrease the mucocilliary clearance (Margerson and Riley, 2003). This, plus the haemodilution from cardiopulmonary bypass, leads to extravascular fluid and the need for patients to have active physiotherapy postoperatively.

- Early ambulation and deep breathing techniques help prevent chest infections. Deep breathing techniques and "huffing" should be taught so the patient can understand and practise these when the physiotherapist is not present. If sputum is purulent, a specimen should be sent for culture and sensitivity.
- Antibiotics should not be given routinely unless the patient presents with other empirical data, for example a raised white cell count and pyrexia.
- Early ambulation also helps to prevent deep vein thrombosis and pulmonary embolism. A low molecular weight heparin should be prescribed daily as prophylaxis and thrombo-embolic stockings should be prescribed, according to the guidleines published by the Department of Health in 2010 (www.dh.gov.uk/en/Publichealth/Healthprotection/Bloodsafety/Venous ThromboembolismVTE/DH_113359).
- Vital signs should be recorded hourly in the immediate postoperative period and reduced to two-hourly then four-hourly as the patient progresses. Four-hourly vital signs should be continued while the patient is hospitalised, as often patients are discharged home on the fourth or fifth postoperative day.
- The majority of patients are only ventilated for a short period of time and can therefore resume their own oral toileting within a few hours, but in patients who are ventilated for more than a few hours oral care is important to prevent ventilator-associated pneumonia (Lorente *et al.*, 2007).

Cardiovascular

Continuous ECG monitoring is carried out in theatre and this should be continued on return to the intensive care unit to observe for arrhythmias. Continuous monitoring of arterial and central venous pressures should also be recommended. The arterial line in the patient's arm should be visible and not hidden by bed sheets so the nurse can observe for signs of bleeding.

There are a number of cardiac complications that can occur after surgery. They may be considered as either pre-cardiac, cardiac or post-cardiac and close observation is required in the 24 hours following surgery.

Pre-cardiac complications

- Hypovolaemia may be classed as a pre-cardiac issue. This may present as hypotension, and a central venous pressure (CVP) reading should then be taken. One lumen of the CVP should be used for measurement only, no other fluid should go through this line as this may give a falsely high reading. Other fluids going through the line may give a falsely high CVP reading. If it is not possible to do this, all other infusions going through the measurement port should be discontinued before a reading is taken. It is advisable not to put other infusions on the line where the CVP is being measured as bolus doses can be given when flushing the line, which can lead to hypotensive or hypertensive crises. If the CVP is low and the hae-moglobin (Hb) is greater than 7 g/dl, crystalloid fluids should be given until the CVP is within normal parameters. If the Hb is less than 6 g/dl and the patient is actively bleeding, blood should be given.

Cardiac complications

Cardiac complications include tamponade, arrhythmias and coronary spasm.

- If the CVP is raised, the urine output is low and the patient is hypotensive, cardiac tamponade should be considered. An urgent chest X-ray may reveal a widened mediastinum, which may be an indicator of tamponade. The treatment for tamponade is to return to theatre for reopening and release of the tamponade. If the patient deteriorates rapidly, emergency reopening in the intensive care unit is indicated.
- Fatal arrhythmias such as asystole and ventricular fibrillation can occur due to the increased secretion of catecholamines resulting from the stress response. Shifts of potassium into the cell may lead to hypokalaemia. For this reason potassium is checked hourly and replacements are given to maintain serum potassium of 4-4.5 mmol/l.
- Coronary artery spasm can occur and presents as ST segment elevation and ventricular arrhythmias (Margerson and Riley, 2003). The treatment for this is a nitroglycerine infusion titrated according to parameters set by the anaesthetist. The guidelines for cardiac arrest post cardiac surgery differ from the Resuscitation Council guidelines and have recently been accepted by the European Association for Cardiac and Thoracic Surgery (Dunning *et al.*, 2009). These recommendations state that in ventricular fibrillation post cardiac surgery, three consecutive shocks should be given before giving cardiac massage or resuscitation drugs. If the shocks are unsuccessful the recommendation is that the patient's chest should be opened as soon as possible in the intensive care unit (Dunning *et al.*, 2009) (*see* Figure 9.1).

CARDIAC ARREST

assess rhythm

ventricular fibrillation or tachycardia	asystole or severe bradycardia	pulseless electrical activity
DC shock (3 attempts)	pace (if wires available)	

start basic life support

amiodarone 300mg via central venous line	atropine 3mg consider external pacing	if paced, turn off pacing to exclude underlying VF

prepare for emergency resternotomy

continue CPR with single DC shock every 2 minutes until resternotomy	continue CPR until resternotomy	continue CPR until resternotomy

airway and ventilation

- If ventilated turn FiO_2 to 100% and switch off PEEP.
- Change to bag/valve with 100% O_2, verify ET tube position and cuff inflation and listen for breath sounds bilaterally to exclude a pneumothorax or haemothorax.
- If tension pneumothorax suspected, immediately place large bore cannula in the 2nd rib space anterior mid-clavicular line.

DO NOT GIVE ADRENALINE unless a senior doctor advises this.

If an IABP is in place change to pressure trigger.

Do not delay basic life support for defibrillation or pacing for more than one minute.

Figure 9.1 Guidelines for resuscitation in cardiac arrest after cardiac surgery. From Dunning *et al.* (2009). Reproduced with permission from Elsevier.

There is a specialist course available that teaches practitioners six key roles to be adopted in the event of an open chest; it has been shown to produce significant improvements in emergency care for patients following cardiac surgery (Dunning *et al.*, 2006) (Figure 9.2).

- Other arrhythmias that may occur are tachyarrhythmias and bradyarrhythmias. A sinus tachycardia is a normal compensatory response and should not be corrected; instead, further investigations should be carried out to determine the cause. Bradycardias can be treated by pacing the patient via temporary wires. Atrial and ventricular temporary wires are often inserted at the end of a cardiac surgical procedure. The most common rhythms requiring pacing include bradycardia, nodal junctional arrhythmias and atrioventricular block.
- Up to four pacing wires can be placed while the patient is in the operating room. Atrial wires are inserted in the right atrial appendage or the body of the right atrium. Ventricular wires are placed on the anterior or diaphragmatic surface of the right ventricle, while the left wire is placed in the apex to the left of the left anterior descending artery or along the obtuse marginal artery. After coronary grafting they are placed behind rather than in front of the saphenous grafts to avoid potential complications relating to graft compression and injury. To determine which wires to attach to the electrodes, remember that atrial wires exit to the left of the midline incision and ventricular wires exit to the right of the midline incision as you look at the patient (Abu-Omar *et al.*, 2006).
- Atrial fibrillation can occur in up to 40% of patients who have had a CABG and up to 60% of patient undergoing valve surgery (Liu and Gropper, 2007) and can be treated with either beta-blockers or amiodarone. The choice of drug is often down to the preference of the surgeon or anaesthetist. Cardioversion can be undertaken in an effort to secure sinus rhythm, as up to 30% of cardiac output can be lost when the synchrony of the heart is disrupted.

Post-cardiac complications

Post-cardiac complications include low output states, vasoplegia and hypertension.

- Low output states also present as hypotension. The definition of a low output syndrome is where the cardiac index is less than 2.4 l/m with evidence of organ dysfunction with either a low urine output or increasing lactate levels (Gillies *et al.*, 2005). Low output states can result in reduced oxygen delivery to vital organs and are therefore important to treat. The use of preoperative angiotension-converting enzyme drugs and opioid anaesthesia are possible causes of postoperative dilatation. Vasoplegia should be ruled out as a cause for the low output.
- In vasoplegia the patient presents with profound dilatation causing a decreased systemic vascular resistance and hypotension. A release of

Figure 3. Six key roles in the cardiac arrest

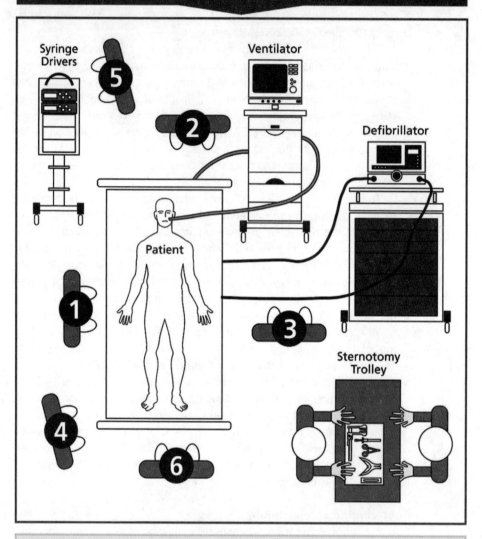

Six key roles in the cardiac arrest:

1. External cardiac massage
2. Airway and breathing
3. Defibrillation
4. Team leader
5. Drugs and syringe drivers
6. ICU co-ordinator

Figure 9.2   The six key roles to be adopted in an intensive care unit when the patient requires emergency re-sternotomy. From Dunning *et al.* (2009). Reproduced with permission from Elsevier.

pro-inflammatory cytokines caused by the cardiopulmonary bypass machine leads to an inflammatory response, which is the major contributory factor (Tripathi *et al.*, 2009). Noradrenaline infusions can be used to treat the vasodilatation by vasoconstriction of the patient. Vasoplegia is not like the normal vasodilatation, which is caused by rewarming the patient after cardiac surgery, which is a gentle process. Bair Huggers can be used to actively warm a profoundly cool patient, and this is especially important if the patient is bleeding. Local protocols are usually developed to guide the use of Bair Huggers. When the patient does not respond to small doses of vasoconstrictors and there is escalation of the noradrenaline infusion it is advisable to get a more accurate measurement of cardiac output. There are various methods for measuring cardiac output, including the oesophageal doppler and the PiCCO (peripherally inserted continuous cardiac output), which is a continuous cardiac output monitoring tool. However, the gold standard remains the pulmonary artery catheter (PAC). A PAC gives an accurate measurement of cardiac output, cardiac index and systemic vascular resistance (SVR). The use of PACs is not without its complications, and these can be fatal. SVR is usually elevated after using the cardiopulmonary bypass machine during surgery because of a transient rise in several vasoconstrictive hormones, including catecholamines, serotonin, arginine and vasopressin. Inodilators such as enoximone and milrinone should be used to treat an elevated SVR with an accompanying hypotension.

- Hypertension can cause disruption of the coronary grafts or cause excessive bleeding from suture lines and should be treated with nitroglycerine infusions and titrated to set parameters for the individual patient.

Cardiac care after the first 24 hours

- The CVP line and arterial line can be removed when the patient is self-ventilating and haemodynamically stable, this is usually on the first post-operative day if there have been no complications. On removing the arterial line firm pressure is needed for at least 5 minutes to ensure bleeding has stopped, although in some cases pressure needs to be administered for longer.
- Patients commonly have excess third space, extravascular fluid in the hands and arms, which eventually absorbs and is helped to disperse with co-amilofruse given postoperatively until the patient reaches their preoperative weight (Olthof *et al.*, 1995).
- As soon as is practicable aspirin and clopidigrel should be either started or recommenced. Warfarin should be commenced for patients who have had mechanical valve replacements. In patients who have had biological valves warfarin is not usually needed, although it may be prescribed if the patient has other high risk factors, for example atrial fibrillation.

Neurological care

Patients are usually sedated with short-acting anaesthetic agents such as propofol while they are mechanically ventilated. This enables the patient to wake quickly once sedation is discontinued (Djaiani et al., 2001).

- The patient's neurological status should be assessed as soon as it is practical following surgery, usually when sedation is being weaned or has been discontinued. The neurological assessment should include pupil size and reaction. Simple commands, for example asking the patients to squeeze your hand and wiggle their toes allows the assessment of their cognitive function and their ability to move their limbs, which also allows assessment of any neurological complications that may have occurred, for example cerebrovascular accidents.
- Sedation should be titrated according to the patient's response to avoid the complications associated with over- and under-sedation. Over-sedation may prolong the period of ventilation and could result in hypotension, which can cause under-perfusion of the coronary grafts; while under-sedation may result in sleep deprivation leading to psychosis or hypertension (caused by an increase in endogenous catecholamines) and/or self-extubation There are many tools available that can be used to assess levels of sedation, and practitioners should decide which tool is the most appropriate for their client group.
- Neurological complications following cardiac surgery range from short-term memory loss to fatal cerebrovascular accidents (Love et al., 2009). Minor complications may not be easily identified by healthcare practitioners, and it is therefore important to involve relatives in assessing patients neurologically as only they may notice subtle changes in patients.

Fluid balance

Intake

Blood transfusion is fairly common after cardiac surgery, with 10–20% of the available blood supply being used in the population of cardiac surgery patients (Surgenor et al., 1992).

- Intraoperative blood salvage and blood sparing interventions should be used to lessen the likelihood of the patient needing blood, for example the use of the cell saver device in theatre.
- Point of care testing should also be available, for example the thromboelastograph, often known as TEG (Sorensen, 2006). This can give information to guide management of blood products and blood transfusions. There are guidelines produced by the Society of Anaesthesiology for the transfusion of packed cells. Transfusion is indicated in patients whose Hb is less than or equal to 6 g/dl, and in whose Hb is 7 g/dl or less and they are older than 65 years or have a chronic cardiovascular or respiratory

condition. In patients whose Hb is 7 to 10 g/dl the benefit of transfusions is unclear. The complications associated with blood transfusion can be fatal (transfusion-related acute lung injury), and this, added to the cost and lack of availability of blood, gives rise to the need for units to produce and follow their own local guidelines based on recommendations.

- While the patient is ventilated acid–base balance should be monitored closely; arterial blood gases also provide information on the acid–base balance. The pH and base deficit should remain within normal parameters. If an acidosis occurs despite correcting any ventilatory problems, meta-bolic causes of acid base imbalances should be explored and treated. Hyperglycaemia should be treated with an insulin infusion. Abdominal causes should be ruled out, as up to 3% of patients undergoing heart surgery suffer from an intra-abdominal complication (Khan *et al.*, 2006).

- Crystalloid such as Hartmann's solution should be given at a rate of 1 ml/ kg/h. In a 70 kg man, 70 ml of crystalloid per hour should be given. If this is given over half an hour it allows enough time for testing of potassium levels before the next infusion is due (Chikwe *et al.*, 2006).

- Anti-emetics should be given for nausea and patients should be encour-aged to take oral fluids and diet as soon as is practicable following removal of the endotracheal tube. Patients should be kept nil by mouth for a short period of time, usually 1 to 2 hours, until it is established that they will not need re-intubating.

Output

Drains should be monitored very closely on return from theatre and should ideally be placed in a position where the nurse can observe them continu-ously. Up to 5 kPa of suction should be connected to drains to aid drainage.

- In the case of bleeding, coagulopathies need to be differentiated from surgical bleeding. Clotting factors (fresh frozen plasma, platelets) and haemostatic drugs (protamine, factor VIIa), may be given to correct coag-ulopathies, while surgical intervention is required if bleeding is from an anastomosis or suture line (Tanos and Dunning, 2006). Drains are usually removed within the first or second postoperative day when drainage has subsided and tied with purse string sutures which are removed anything between 4 and 10 days after drain removal.

- A urinary catheter is inserted while the patient is in theatre, after induc-tion, and the goal is 1 ml/kg. Urine output is indicative of end organ func-tion, which is indicative of a failing cardiac output. Urine output should be monitored hourly and should be no less than 0.5 ml/kg. If it falls below this level intervention is needed.

- Bowel function should have returned to normal within 2 days of surgery. Laxatives can be prescribed if normal bowel function has not returned.

Skin integrity

There are a number of categories of patient who are at increased risk of pressure ulcer development after cardiac surgery.

- Patients who have had a long bypass time.
- Patients who have diabetes mellitus.
- Patients with low preoperative haemoglobin level.
- Patients with low albumin levels.
- Patients who have an intra-aortic balloon pump in situ.
- Patients who are turned less often.
- Patients who have a more rapid return to preoperative body temperature (Pokony et al., 2003; Lewicki et al., 1997).

Nurses should be vigilant in their observation of skin integrity and the patient should be repositioned two- to four-hourly when their haemodynamic condition allows. As well as observation of the sacrum, care should be taken with patients' heels, especially when they have an intra-aortic balloon pump in situ. Wound dressings should be removed 48 hours after surgery and left uncovered if there is no exudate.

Pain control

While patients are ventilated and sedated it is important to ensure adequate pain relief is given. Intravenous paracetamol and/or opiate infusions should be titrated according to the patient's vital signs. In patients who are sedated, assessment of pain should include signs of catecholamine release where hypertension and tachycardia are present, as this may be the only indicator of pain. When patients are self-ventilating and able to take oral medication, oral analgesia should be prescribed and given according to the patient's self-reported pain scores.

Psychological care

Post-cardiotomy delirium (PCD) is a serious event that results in higher morbidity and mortality rates, and prolonged hospitalisation (Giltay et al., 2006). Some variables that have been identified which seem to have a crucial role in the aetiology of delirium after cardiac surgery are:

- perioperative hypoxia
- anaemia
- preoperative psychiatric disorders such as depression and cognitive impairment
- alcohol use in the week before surgery (Kazmierski et al., 2008).

Patients who develop PCD usually require drug therapy to control the delirium, although in mild cases it is possible for a full recovery with no drug intervention. Haloperidol is often used to treat this condition.

Antimicrobial therapy

Prophylactic antibiotics are given pre-procedure and-post procedure because of the highly invasive nature of the surgery. Local guidelines are established on how many doses and which antibiotics are given. It is common in the first few hours after surgery for the patient to have pyrexias. These should not be treated unless they persist and should not be taken as a sign of infection. After 24–48 hours if a pyrexia is persistent, the patient should be screened for infection and treated appropriately.

Fast tracking

Historically, patients were nursed in intensive care and ventilated over-night following all cardiac surgical procedures, but practice has changed dramatically since the mid-1980s.The concept of fast tracking of patients is now performed in most centres. Some centres have specific short stay areas while other centres fast track the patient through an intensive care bed, then move the patient to a lower dependency bed in another area.

The widely accepted definition of fast track is the cessation of mechanical ventilation and extubation 1–6 hours after surgery (Cheng, 1998). Guidelines based on physiology-bound protocols are used on the basis of specific body parameters as opposed to the traditionally used time course. Fast tracking patients has been found to reduce mortality and some of the complications related to extended intubation times, for example infections, anxiety and psychosis (Engoren, 1998).

The necessary elements required for effective fast tracking are:

- patient selection
- titration of short-acting anaesthetic drugs
- standardised surgical procedures
- early extubation
- rewarming with sustained postoperative normothermia
- good postoperative pain control
- early ambulation and discharge.

Propofol has become the major component of fast track and in cardiac anaesthesia it is widely used for induction due to its short half life (Djaiani et al., 2001).

As well as the benefits for the patient, fast tracking also shortens the period of time in the critical care unit and the overall length of stay for the patient. It impacts beneficially on operative cancellation rates and frees up intensive care beds for emergencies (Aps, 2006). This obviously impacts on the cost of the service, which places less stress on the National Health Service per se (Engelman et al., 1994).

Discharge

All wounds should be checked on the day of discharge for signs of infection, and district nurses should be booked if the patient needs further observation. Pacing wires should be removed either on the day of discharge or the day before. This should be done while the patient is on a bed and they should be asked to rest for at least one hour after removal. The patient should be observed and vital signs recorded to exclude a cardiac tamponade or disruption of the grafts.

Patients should be given advice on:

- diet
- exercise
- resumption of sexual activity
- driving
- travelling
- increasing activity levels gradually and cardiac rehabilitation
- activities that should not be undertaken
- care of the wounds
- medications.

They should also be provided with information booklets that reiterate the advice given. All medications should be explained, including why they have been prescribed and what they for. Follow-up appointments should be made and contact numbers given in case the patient has any queries.

Summary

The nurse plays a major role in stabilising the haemodynamic status of the patient following cardiac surgery, and it takes an in-depth knowledge of physiology and clinical experience to care for this group of patients. The development of individual assessment skills is paramount, as it is often the nurse who leads patient progress, and makes decisions based on this, within the cardiothoracic intensive care area. Therefore the development of finely tuned assessment skills is paramount. Many nurses have enhanced their roles to include areas such as weaning patients from ventilation. The reduction in junior doctors' hours means new roles are being developed for nurses, and they may now manage the entire episode of care for patients, from running preadmission clinics, to the immediate postoperative period and up to and including discharge.

References

Abu-Omar Y and Taggart DP (2009) The present status off-pump coronary artery grafting. *European Journal of Cardiothoracic Surgery* **36**: 312-21.

Antunes PE, Ferrão de Oliveira J and Antunes MJ (2009) Risk-prediction for postoperative major morbidity in coronary surgery. *European Journal of Cardiothoracic Surgery* **35**: 760-7.

Aps C (2006) Adopting a fast track approach to cardiac surgery. *British Journal of Cardiac Nursing* **1**(4): 175-9.

Cahill RA, McGreal GT and Crowe BH (2005) Duration of increased bleeding tendency after cessation of aspirin therapy. *Journal of the American College of Surgeons* **4**: 564-73.

Cheng D (1998) Fast track cardiac surgery pathways. Early extubation, process of care and cost containment. *Anesthesiology* **88**(6): 1429-33.

Chikwe J, Beddow E and Glenville B (2006) *Cardiothoracic Surgery. Oxford Specialist Handboook in Surgery.* Oxford, Oxford University Press.

Coggon J (2008) Arterial blood gas analysis 1. *Understanding ABG Reports* **104**(18): 28-9.

Department of Health (2001) *National Service Framework for the Older Person.* London, Department of Health.

Djaiani GN, Hall J, Pugh S and Peaston RT (2001) Vital capacity inhalation induction with sevoflurane: an alternative to standard induction with sevoflurane IV induction for patients undergoing cardiac surgery. *Journal of Cardiovascular Anesthesiology* **15**: 169-74.

Dunning J, Fabbri A, Kolh PH *et al.* (2009) Guideline for resuscitation in cardiac arrest after cardiac surgery *European Journal of Cardiothoracic Surgery* **36**: 3-28.

Dunning J, Nandi J, Ariffin S, Jerstice J, Danitsch D and Levine A (2006) The cardiac surgery advanced life support course (CALS): delivering significant improvement in emergency cardiothoracic care. *Annals of Thoracic Surgery* **81**(1): 1767-72.

Engelman RM, Rousou JA and Flack JE (1994) Fast track recovery of the coronary artery bypass graft patient. *Annals of Thoracic Surgery* **58**: 1742-6.

Engoren MC, Kraras C and Gazia F (1998) Propofol based versus fentanyl isoflurane base anaesthesia for cardiac surgery. *Journal of Cardiothoracic and Vascular Anaesthesia* **12**: 177-81.

Germing A and Mügge A (2009) What the cardiac surgeon needs to know prior to aortic valve surgery: impact of echocardiography. *European Journal of Cardiothoracic Surgery* **35**: 960-4.

Gillies M, Bellomo R, Doolan L and Buxton B (2005) Bench to bedside review:inotropic drug therapy after adult cardiac surgery – a systematic literature review. *Critical Care* **9**: 266-79.

Giltay EJ, Huijskes RVHP, King H, Kho KH, Blansjaar BA and Rosseel PMJ (2006) Psychotic symptoms in patients undergoing coronary artery bypass grafting and heart valve operation. *European Journal of Cardiothoracic Surgery* **30**: 140-7.

Kazmierski J, Kowman M, Banach M *et al.* (2008) Clinical utility and use of DSM-IV and ICD-10 criteria and the memorial delirium assessment scale in establishing a diagnosis of delirium after cardiac surgery. *Psychomatics* **49**(1): 73-6.

Khan JH, Lambert AM, Habib JH, Broce M, Emmett MS and Davis EA (2006) Abdominal Complications After Heart Surgery. *Annals of Thoracic Surgery* **82**(5): 1796-801.

Lewicki LJ, Mion L, Splane G, Samstas D and Secic M (1997) Patients risk factors for pressure ulcers during cardiac surgery. *Association of Perioperative Registered Nurses* **65**(5): 933-42.

Lewis ME, Al-Khalidi AH, Townend JN, Cooke J and Bonser RS (2002) The effects of hypothermia on human left ventricular contractile function during cardiac surgery. *Journal of American College of Cardiology* **39**: 102-8.

Liu LL and Gropper MA (2007) Respiratory and haemodynamic management after cardiac surgery. *Current Treatment Options in Cardiovascular Medicine* **4**(2): 161-9.

Lorente L, Blot S and Rello J (2007) Evidence on measures for the prevention of ventilator-associated pneumonia. *European Respiratory Journal* **30**(6): 1193-207.

Love B, Hocker SE and Biller J (2009) on www.medlink.com/medlinkcontent.asp (accessed 20 April 2010)

Mangano DT (2002) Aspirin and mortality from coronary bypass surgery. *New England Journal of Medicine* **347**(17): 1309-17.

Margerson C and Riley J (2003) *Cardiothoracic Surgical Nursing. Current Trends in Adult Care.* Oxford, Blackwell Science.

Mosteller RD (1987) Simplified calculation of body surface area. *New England Journal of Medicine* **317**: 1098.

Myles PS, Buckland MR and Weeks AM (1997) Haemodynamic effects, myocardial ischaemia and timing of tracheal extubation with propofol based anesthesia for cardiac surgery. *Anaesthetic Analgesia* **84**: 12-19.

Ning XH, Xu CS, Song YC *et al.* (1998) Hypothermia preserves functional signalling for mitochondria biogenesis duing subsequent ischaemia in isolated rabbit heart. *American Journal of Physiology of the Heart and Ciculatory Physiology* **274**: 786-93.

Olthof CG, Jansen PGM, De Vries JPPM *et al.* (1995) Interstitial fluid volume during cardiac surgery measured by means of a non invasive conductivity technique. *Acta Anaestesiological Scandinavia* **39**(4): 505-12.

Pedro EA, Ferrão H, de Oliveira M and Antunes J (2009) Risk-prediction for postoperative major morbidity in coronary surgery. *European Journal of Cardiothoracic Surgery* **35**: 760-7.

Pokony ME, Koljeski D and Swanson M (2003) Skin care interventions for patients having cardiac surgery. *American Journal of Critical Care* **12**: 535-44.

Sorensen ER (2006) Imrove cardiac outcomes with TEG. *Nursing Critical Care* **1**(2): 18-24.

Surgenor DM, Wallace EL, Churchill WH, Hao SH, Chapman RH and Collins Jr JJ (1992) Red cell transfusion in coronary artery bypass graft surgery. *Transfusion* **32**: 458-64.

Tanos M and Dunning J (2006) Is recombinant activated factor VIIa useful for intractable bleeding after cardiac surgery? *European Association of Cardiothoracic surgery. Interactive Cardiovascular and Thoracic Surgery.* http://icvts.ctsnetjournals.org/cgi/content/full/5/4/493 (accessed 20 January 2010).

Tonz M, Mihaljevic T, von Segesser LK *et al.* (1995) normothermia versus hypo-thermia during cardiopulmonary bypass: a randomised controlled trial. *Annals of Thoracic Surgery* **59**: 137-43.

Tripathi M, Singh PK, Kumar N and Pant KC (2009) Induced mild hypothermia in post cardiopulmonary bypass vasoplegia syndrome. *Annals of Cardiac Anaesthesia* **12**(1): 49-52.

Web resources

www.dh.gov.uk/en/Publichealth/Healthprotection/Bloodsafety/VenousThromboembolismVTE/DH_113359 (accessed on 20 April 2010).

www.library.nhs.uk/theatres/viewResource.aspx?resid=259250&code=60aa705 0a268a407c3333b03437d2799 (accessed on 20 April 2010).

www.mpoullis.com/euro.htm (accessed on 20 April 2010).

www.scts.org/documents/PDF/BCISTAVIDec2008.pdf (accessed on 19 January 2010).

Chapter 10

Arrhythmias and their Management

Melanie Humphreys, Celia Warlow and John McGowan

Introduction

Cardiac arrhythmia is a generic term used for any of a heterogeneous group of conditions in which there is abnormal electrical activity in the heart. Some arrhythmias may cause only irritating symptoms such as an awareness of the heart beating very fast, others may cause potentially life-threatening conditions such as a stroke or cardiac arrest.

Normal sinus rhythm is the natural rhythm of the heart. Synchronous contraction of the atria, followed by that of the ventricles optimises blood flow. If the heart rate is too fast or too slow, insufficient blood may be pumped to meet the demands of the organs of the body. The aim of this chapter is to gain an understanding of the manifestations and mechanisms of arrhythmias, in order to enhance confidence when nursing patients who may experience cardiac arrhythmias.

> ### Learning outcomes
>
> At the end of the chapter, the reader will be able to:
>
> - discuss the main aspects of the electrophysiology of the heart and their relationship to the conduction system
> - discuss in detail the common bradyarrhythmias and tachyarrhythmias and outline their likely management
> - describe how to recognise cardiac arrest, what rhythms this may encompass, and its management.

Nursing the Cardiac Patient, First Edition. Edited by Melanie Humphreys.
© 2011 Blackwell Publishing Ltd. Published 2011 by Blackwell Publishing Ltd.

Electrophysiology of the heart

Each cardiac muscle cell or myocyte is, in common with other muscle cells and neurons, polarised at rest. That is, the inside of the cell has a negative voltage compared with the outside. This is maintained by the relative ion concentrations in the two areas. Inside the cell, potassium concentrations are high and sodium concentrations low, whereas outside the cell, potassium concentrations are low and sodium high. The cell membrane allows sodium to pass through readily, so the low levels of sodium inside the cell are dependent on ion pumps, fuelled by ATP.

When stimulated, usually by the depolarisation of an adjacent myocyte, electrical channels open in the cell membrane, allowing rapid changes in the ion concentrations. This depolarisation produces the action potential, essentially a graph of the voltage changes in the cell against time (Figure 10.1)

The five phases of the action potential in Figure 10.1 are as follows.

- *Phase 4* - the resting phase. The cell is negatively charged compared with the outside. This difference, of about 85 mV, is called the resting membrane potential. Potassium is high inside and sodium is high outside the cell.
- *Phase 0* - except in the sinoatrial (SA) and atrioventricular (AV) nodes, the cells rapidly depolarise. Channels on the cell membrane open and sodium ions enter. This changes the cell's negative electrical charge to a positive one as it depolarises.
- *Phase 1* - the cells rapidly repolarise. This is caused by fast sodium channels closing and by potassium leaving the cell.
- *Phase 2* - the action potential reaches a plateau, as the cell's electrical activity stabilises. Calcium flows into and potassium flows out of the cell.
- *Phase 3* - the cell completes repolarisation. Ion pumps move sodium out and potassium into the cell. When the cell's membrane potential drops, the absolute refractory period ends and the relative refractory period begins.

The speed with which cells depolarise depends on whether a fast or slow channel dominates them. Fast and slow channels are the routes through

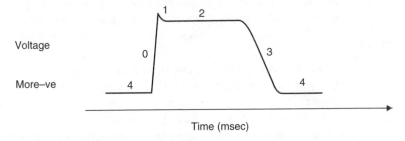

Figure 10.1 Cardiac action potential.

which sodium and calcium flow in and out of the cell. If the fast channel dominates, the cell depolarises quickly. Conversely, if the slow channel dominates, the cell depolarises slowly. Fast channels dominate cardiac muscle cells, while slow channels dominate cardiac electrical cells. It is also of note that each action potential lasts about one thousandth of a second.

Refractory period

This is the time it takes after depolarisation for the cell to depolarise in response to a second stimulus. Referring to the action potential above, in phase 2, no stimulus will cause depolarisation. In phase 3, a stronger than usual stimulus will depolarise the membrane; however, there is a short period during phase 3, the supranormal period, when a weaker than usual impulse may cause depolarisation (Grant and Durrani, 2007). The refractory period gives direction to impulse propagation: the cell that has just stimulated depolarisation in a second cell cannot be stimulated to depolarise by the second cell, as it will be refractory.

As stated earlier, myocyte depolarisation may be triggered by depolarisation of an adjacent cell, which would effectively mean that a wave of depolarisation would spread like a ripple across the myocardium. This is prevented by intercellular proteins called connexins, which channel these depolarisations through tracts in the myocardium.

Depolarisation of the cell membrane changes the concentration of calcium and other intracellular messengers that activate contraction of the myocardial cell.

The depolarisation/repolarisation of the millions of cells in the heart can be measured on the body surface and are what produces the electrocardiogram (ECG).

The conduction system

The normal heartbeat originates from spontaneously depolarising cells in an area of tissue in the right atrium of the heart, the sinoatrial (SA) node. The rate at which these cells depolarise is influenced by sympathetic and parasympathetic activity. Sympathetic stimulation increases this rate; parasympathetic (vagal) stimulation decreases the rate at which these cells depolarise.

Depolarisation of the SA node depolarises adjacent cells and a wave of depolarisation spreads across the atria, causing atrial contraction. Inside the right atrium, close to the tricuspid valve, is another area of specialised conductive tissue, the atrioventricular (AV) node. This has the lowest conduction velocity in the myocardium. This slows transmission of atrial depolarisation to the ventricles.

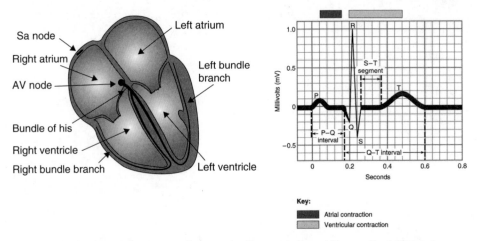

Sa node
Right atrium
AV node
Bundle of his
Right ventricle
Right bundle branch

Left atrium
Left bundle branch
Left ventricle

Figure 10.2 The cardiac conduction system and its manifestation into the QRS complex. P wave – atrial systole; PR interval – delay at the AV node; QRS complex – ventricular systole; T wave – ventricular repolarisation.

The impulse then spreads through both ventricles via the right and left bundle branches and the Purkinje fibres, causing a synchronised contraction of the heart muscle (Figure 10.2).

Re-entry phenomena

Many arrhythmias are caused by re-entrant excitation. These are due to lack of homogeneity in the conduction of impulses within the myocardium, which can have a number of causes including, ischaemia, stretch and scarring. This phenomenon is illustrated in Figure 10.3 (adapted from Hoffman and Rosen, 1981).

Manifestations of arrhythmias

The best way of diagnosing any arrhythmia is by medical assessment, including an electrocardiogram (ECG) (Schamroth, 1990). The clinical importance of an arrhythmia in a patient is related to the ventricular rate, the presence of any underlying heart disease and the reliability of cardiovascular reflexes.

Coronary blood flow occurs during diastole, and as the heart rate increases, the diastolic period shortens. In the patient with coronary heart disease, blood flow in the coronary arteries can be reduced and chest pain may occur. Reduced cardiac performance produces symptoms of faintness or syncope and leads to increased sympathetic stimulation, which may increase the heart rate even further.

An ECG is important in the assessment of the patient for determining the heart rhythm and how to proceed with the nursing management. The ECG transforms the electrical activity it picks up from each lead into a series of

(a)

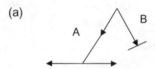

(b)

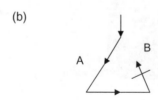

(c)

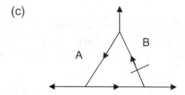

Figure 10.3 (a) Depolarisation spreads down paths A and B. In path A it continues on to other tissues. However, in path B, the depolarisation is blocked. (b) Depolarisation continues retrogradely in path B, but is not blocked in this direction. (c) The re-entrant circuit is complete. Other tissue, adjacent to the re-entry circuit is depolarised much more quickly than it would be by normal conduction.

waveforms, which correspond to depolarisation and repolarisation within the heart (Figure 10.4).

- *P wave* - represents the time necessary for an electrical impulse to spread throughout the atrial musculature.
- *PR interval* - measures the spread of the impulse through the AV node. It is measured from the beginning of the QRS complex. Normal duration ranges from 0.12 to 0.20 s.
- *QRS complex* - normally has a greater amplitude than the P wave because ventricular muscle mass is greater than atrial. Normal duration is up to 0.10 s. Deflections of the QRS complex vary according to whether the electrical activity is travelling towards the positive electrode or away from it. When electrical activity travels towards the positive electrode, a positive deflection is seen. Conversely, when it travels towards the negative electrode, a negative deflection is seen. The first negative deflection is called the Q wave. The first positive deflection is called the R wave and the downward deflection following is called the S wave. The QRS complex can take on many different configurations, which can be normal.
- *ST segment* - no electrical activity occurs at this time, and therefore the ST segment remains at the baseline or isoelectric line. It is normally between 0.08 and 0.12 s.

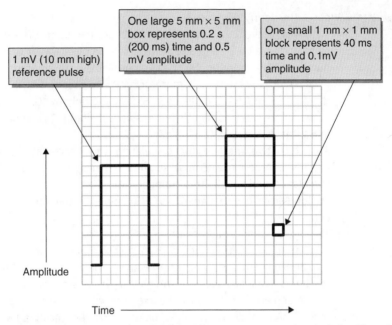

One large 5 mm × 5 mm box represents 0.2 s (200 ms) time and 0.5 mV amplitude

One small 1 mm × 1 mm block represents 40 ms time and 0.1mV amplitude

1 mV (10 mm high) reference pulse

Amplitude

Time

Figure 10.4 ECG paper: one large 5 mm square represents 0.2 s. Therefore five large squares represent 1 s in time.

- *T wave* – the peak of the T wave represents the vulnerable period of repolarisation. At this time a weak electrical stimulus can precipitate depolarisation and therefore can cause serious arrhythmias.
- *QT interval* – this includes the QRS complex, ST segment and the T wave. Normal QT intervals vary from patient to patient, with variants including age and sex. It varies between 0.30 and 0.45 s and it will shorten as the heart rate increases. For this reason, the corrected QT interval (QTc) is used. This is calculated using the formula

$$QTc = \frac{QT}{\sqrt{(\text{R-R interval in seconds})}}$$

Most ECG machines do this calculation automatically and the QTc should be 0.38–0.42 s.

Questions to ask when diagnosing a rhythm

- Is there electrical activity?
  - If there is no electrical activity, check the leads, electrical connections and gain on the machine. If there is still no electrical activity, the rhythm is asystole.
  - If electrical activity is present, check to see if there are recognisable complexes. If there are none, the rhythm may be ventricular fibrillation, which presents as a rapid, bizarre, irregular appearance with random frequency.
  - If there are recognisable complexes, go to the next question.

- What is the ventricular rate?
  - A normal resting heart rate is 60-100 beats/min (bpm). The ventricular rate can be calculated in a few ways. The simplest way is to record the number on the monitor. This can be unreliable if the rhythm is irregular or artefact is present. It is more accurate to record a strip and count the number of QRS complexes in 6s and multiply by 10. This gives the approximate rate per minute. For example, if eight QRS complexes occur in 6s, the rate is $8 \times 10 = 80$/min.
  - An alternative method for calculating the heart rate is to count the number of large (5mm) squares between two consecutive QRS complexes and divide this number into 300. For example, if there are four large boxes between two QRS complexes, the rate is 300/4 = 75/min.
- Is the QRS rhythm regular or irregular?
  - Look at an adequate length of rhythm strip and measure out the intervals between R waves. The interval should be fairly regular. If the QRS rhythm is irregular, decide if the basic rhythm is regular with intermittent irregularity or if it is totally irregular with no recognisable pattern of R-R interval. There may also be a recurring cyclical variation in the R-R intervals (Table 3.4).
- Is the QRS width normal or prolonged?
  - A normal QRS complex should be 0.12s (three small boxes) or less. This indicates the impulse has originated above the ventricles and may be from the SA node, atria or AV node.
  - If the QRS duration is >0.12s, the rhythm may be originating in the ventricular myocardium or may be a supraventricular rhythm.
- Is atrial activity present?
  - After determining the rate, regularity and QRS width, look to see if there are any identifiable P waves. This may be difficult either because the P waves are too small or because the atrial activity is partly or fully obscured by QRS complexes or T waves. Sinus P waves are usually seen best in lead II.
  - Other types of atrial activity may be present. Atrial flutter waves occur when the atrium are depolarising at a rapid rate. The waves have a classic "saw tooth" pattern, often at a rate of 300/min.
  - Atrial fibrillation happens when the waves of depolarisation happen randomly through both atria. There are no P waves. AF waves are usually seen as rapid deviations from the ECG baseline with varying size and duration.
- How is atrial activity related to ventricular activity?
  - A consistent interval between P waves and the following QRS complex indicates that conduction between the atrium and ventricle is intact. The interval between atrial depolarisation and ventricular depolarisation is referred to as the P-R interval and is normally 0.12-0.20s (three to five small boxes). Occasionally, there are conduction problems between the atria and ventricles and a number of arrhythmias may arise (Table 3.4).

It is helpful to remember that effective treatment is often possible without a precise ECG diagnosis and the full clinical assessment must be considered; these basic questions will help to identify the patient's rhythm and its origin. They facilitate a systematic approach to analysing the rhythm.

Arrhythmias

In adults, a bradycardia is defined as a ventricular rate of less than 60 bpm; a tachycardia is a rate greater than 100 bpm. With all the given rhythm strips, attempt to work out the heart rate using the calculation example given. What follows is not an exhaustive list, rather the arrhythmias more commonly encountered.

Bradyarrhythmias

Sinus bradycardia (Figure 10.5)

The heart rate is slower than normal; however, the pattern remains the same. It is usually benign and results from a good general fitness level or drugs such as beta-blockers.

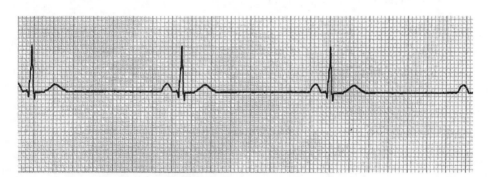

Figure 10.5 Sinus bradycardia.

What is the QRS rate?	Less than 60 bpm
Is the QRS rhythm regular?	Yes
What is the QRS duration?	Less than 0.12 s (three small squares)
Is there atrial activity?	P waves
Are there P waves before each QRS?	Yes
What is the PR interval?	0.12–0.20 s (three to five small squares)

Atrioventricular (AV) blocks

The SA node may be generating impulses causing the atria to contract at a normal rate, but not every impulse passes through the AV node to the ventricles. Heart blocks may be congenital or acquired, for example following an ischaemic event. There are various types of AV block.

First degree AV block (Figure 10.6)

This is simply a delay in conduction through the conducting system. It is diagnosed by a prolonged PR interval, beyond the normal 0.20 s. Importantly, each P wave is followed by a QRS complex.

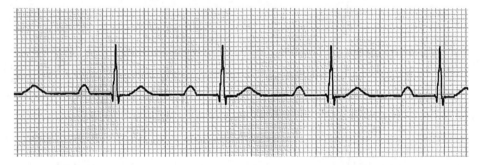

Figure 10.6   First degree AV block.

What is the QRS rate?	Dependent on the underlying rhythm
Is the QRS rhythm regular?	Yes
What is the QRS duration?	Less than 0.12 s (three small squares)
Is there atrial activity?	Yes, P waves
Are there P waves before each QRS?	Yes
What is the PR interval?	Greater than 0.20 s (five small squares)

Second degree AV block

Here, the rhythm is characterised by an intermittent failure or interruption of AV node conduction. The P wave is blocked within the AV conducting system, and in effect is "dropped" and hence not followed by a QRS complex.

- *Second degree AV block* (Mobitz type 1 – Wenkebach phenomenon) (Figure 10.7) Cellular depolarisation in the AV node becomes more prolonged, usually due to ischaemia in these tissues. As a result, the refractory period is prolonged. On the surface ECG, this rhythm has an initially normal PR interval, with each subsequent PR interval becoming more prolonged. The cycle is complete when atrial activation occurs while the AV node is refractory, and no ventricular conduction occurs, resulting in a "dropped" QRS complex. The PR interval following the dropped beat will be normal, as AV nodal tissue will have recovered. The sequence then continues to repeat itself.

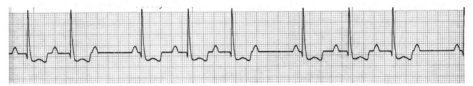

Figure 10.7   Second degree AV block, type 1.

What is the QRS rate?	Ventricular is usually slower than the atrial rate
Is the QRS rhythm regular?	No
What is the QRS duration?	Less than 0.12 s (three small squares)
Is there atrial activity?	Yes
Are there P waves before each QRS?	Yes, but some P waves are not followed by a QRS.
What is the PR interval?	Progressively lengthening until a QRS is "dropped"

- *2:1 AV block*   (Figure 10.8) This is probably a short-cycle Wenkebach-type block. The QRS complexes are usually narrow, but there are two P waves for every QRS complex.

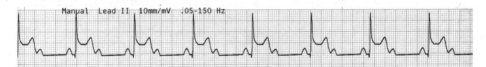

Manual   Lead II   10mm/mV   .05-150 Hz

Figure 10.8   2:1 AV block.

What is the QRS rate?	Slow
Is the rhythm regular?	Yes
What is the QRS duration?	Usually Less than 0.12 s (three small squares)
Is there atrial activity?	Yes, P waves
Are there P waves before each QRS?	Yes, but every second P wave is not followed by a QRS complex
What is the PR interval?	Normal for conducted beats

- *Second degree AV block*   (Mobitz type 2) (Figure 10.9) In this type of block the PR interval is usually normal, but the QRS complexes are prolonged. There are intermittent dropped beats, often with two or three P waves not conducted to the ventricles. The conduction abnormality arises in the bundle of His and the bundle branches. This rhythm carries a risk of progression to complete heart block or ventricular asystole (Narula and Samet, 1970).

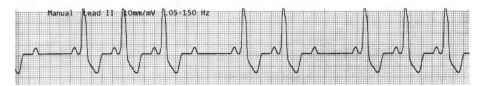

Figure 10.9 Second degree AV block, type 2.

What is the QRS rate?	May be normal
Is the QRS rhythm regular?	No
What is the QRS duration?	Greater than 0.12 s (three small squares)
Is there atrial activity?	Yes, P waves
Are there P waves before each QRS?	Yes, but some P waves are not followed by a QRS
What is the PR interval?	Less than 0.20 s for conducted beats

● *Third degree AV block* (complete heart block) (Figure 10.10) This is characterised by complete interruption of conduction between the atria and
ventricles. All impulses from the atria are blocked below the AV node,
allowing the atria and ventricles to beat independently (Wolbrette and
Nacarelli, 2007). A secondary pacemaker stimulates the ventricles and the
ventricular rate will be dependent on the site of the secondary pacemaker.
If it is situated around the AV node, the QRS rate may be near to normal
and the complexes of normal duration. However, if the secondary pacemaker is located within the ventricle, the QRS complex will be widened
and the ventricular rate slower (20–40 bpm).

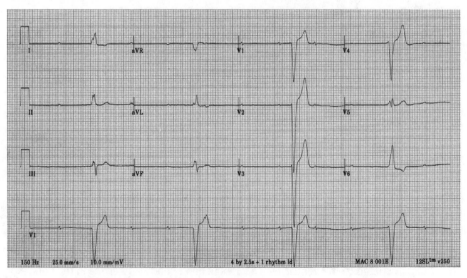

Figure 10.10 Third degree AV block.

What is the QRS rate?	Slow
Is the QRS rhythm regular?	Yes
What is the QRS duration?	Dependent on pacemaker site: close to the AV node, normal. Within the ventricles, wide
Is there atrial activity?	Yes
Are there P waves before each QRS?	Unrelated. More P waves than QRS complexes
What is the PR interval?	Variable

Tacharrhythmias

Sinus tachycardia (Figure 10.11)

The heart rate is faster than normal. It is usually a physiological response but may be precipitated by certain drugs or endocrine disturbances. Each P wave is followed by a QRS complex. The rate rarely exceeds 180 bpm.

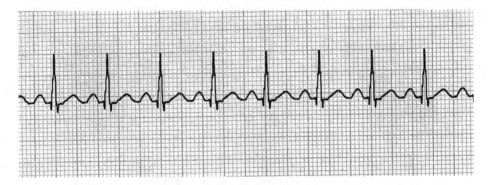

Figure 10.11 Sinus tachycardia.

What is the QRS rate?	100-180 bpm
Is the QRS rhythm regular?	Yes
What is the QRS duration?	Usually less than 0.12 s (three small squares)
Is there atrial activity?	Yes
Are there P waves before each QRS?	Yes
What is the PR interval?	0.12-0.20 s (three to five small squares)

Atrial fibrillation (AF) (Figure 10.12)

This is a common arrhythmia, present in 0.4-1% of the population. It becomes more common with increasing age and can be difficult to treat (Fuster *et al.*, 2006). The longer a patient has been in AF, the more likely electrical remodelling will occur, where changes in the conductivity and in the action potential of atrial cells makes restoration of sinus rhythm less likely. In AF, depolarisation occurs in multiple wavelets throughout the atria (Cobbe and Rankin,

1993). Instead of contracting rhythmically, the atria quiver and depolarisation of the AV node occurs at frequent and irregular intervals. The surface ECG shows no organised P waves, but irregular activity on the baseline, called F waves. Because there is no organised atrial contraction, small blood clots can form on the atrial wall. These are the main cause of the increased stroke risk in patients with atrial fibrillation.

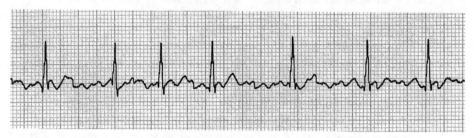

Figure 10.12   Atrial fibrillation.

What is the QRS rate?	May be normal, slow or fast
Is the QRS rhythm regular?	No
What is the QRS duration?	Usually less than 0.12 s (three small squares)
Is there atrial activity?	Yes, F waves
Are there P waves before each QRS?	No
What is the PR interval?	There is no P wave

Atrial flutter (Figure 10.13)

This is typically caused by a large re-entry circuit in the right atrium. This depolarises the atria at rates between 250 and 350 times per minute (Blomstrom-Lindqvist *et al.*, 2003). The slowly conducting AV node is unable to depolarise at this rate, so ventricular activation is much slower. Atrial flutter is often expressed as a ratio of atrial to ventricular rate, e.g. a 3:1 conduction means that every third atrial impulse is conducted to the ventricles. The rapid atrial depolarisation is seen on the surface ECG as flutter waves, which may be "saw tooth" in appearance in some leads. The QRS rhythm may be regular or irregular, depending on AV nodal conduction. Typically the QRS duration is normal as the impulses arise from above the His bundle.

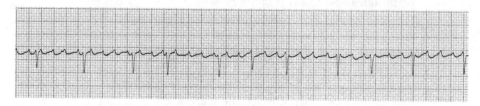

Figure 10.13   Atrial flutter.

What is the QRS rate?	May be normal or rapid
Is the QRS rhythm regular?	May be regular or irregular
What is the QRS duration?	Usually less than 0.12 s (three small squares)
Is there atrial activity?	Yes, regular, rapid flutter waves often 300/min (one large square apart)
Are there P waves before each QRS?	More flutter waves than QRS complexes
What is the PR interval?	Variable

Supraventricular tachycardia (SVT) (Figure 10.14)

This is a bit of a catch-all term for a number of different tachycardias origi-nating above the His bundle. Any fast rhythm that activates the His-Purkinje system in the normal way and therefore produces a narrow QRS complex gives an "SVT". SVT can be caused by re-entry circuits involving the AV node directly or through accessory pathways connecting the atrium and ventri-cles; it can also be produced by any focal atrial arrhythmia or re-entrant circuit within the atria. Normally SVT is remarkably well tolerated despite ventricular rates, which can reach 280/min.

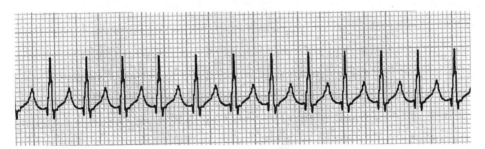

Figure 10.14 Supraventricular tachycardia.

What is the QRS rate?	150–250 bpm. It is worth noting that there are some SVTs that can go as fast as 320 bpm if there is abnormal AV node physiology (but this is extremely rare). 1:1 conducted atrial flutter can also cause a rate in excess of 300 bpm
Is the QRS rhythm regular?	Yes
What is the QRS duration?	Normally less than 0.12 s (three small squares)
Is there atrial activity?	Yes, but may not be discernable at faster rates
Are there P waves before each QRS?	Yes, but may not be discernable at faster rates
What is the PR interval?	May be shorter than normal (less than three small squares)

Sick sinus syndrome

This the general term used for a variety of arrhythmias including profound bradycardias, bradycardias which don't respond to exercise, sinus arrest and paroxysmal tachycardias including AF. The syndrome occurs mainly, but not exclusively, in the elderly and is thought to be due to degenerative fibrosis in the SA node (Dobrzynski et al., 2007). Some familial forms may be due to genetic variation in ion channels in the SA node. Treatment is by permanent pacing, with anti-arrhythmic drugs to suppress tachyarrhythmias and anti-coagulation for AF.

Life-threatening arrhythmias

Ventricular tachycardia (monomorphic VT) (Figure 10.15)

This is caused by single or multiple re-entrant circuits within the ventricles. It is defined as three or more consecutive ventricular beats at a rate greater than 120/min (Cobbe and Rankin, 1993). At slower rates, VT may be well tolerated. However, it may cause syncope or cardiac arrest. In the absence of a pulse or other signs of life, the patient should be defibrillated as soon as possible, and cardiopulmonary resuscitation (CPR) should be performed until this can be done. VT may deteriorate into ventricular fibrillation; however, the mechanism for this is unclear (Samie and Jose, 2001).

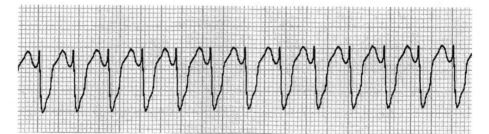

Figure 10.15   Ventricular tachycardia.

What is the QRS rate?	Greater than 120 bpm
Is the QRS rhythm regular?	Yes
What is the QRS duration?	Prolonged, greater than 0.12 s (three small squares)
Is there atrial activity?	P waves may occasionally seen
Are there P waves before each QRS?	No
What is the PR interval?	Variable

Torsades de pointes (polymorphic VT) (Figure 10.16)

In this variant ventricular tachycardia, each QRS complex is a different shape to the one preceding it, the net effect on the surface ECG being that the QRS complex appears to twist around the baseline. The QRS complexes are bizarre and multiform, with the sharp points directed one way for a few seconds and then directed in another way, hence the term (Schamroth, 1990). As with monomorphic VT, this arrhythmia may cause syncope or cardiac arrest. It is a rare arrhythmia, and may be caused by QT prolongation.

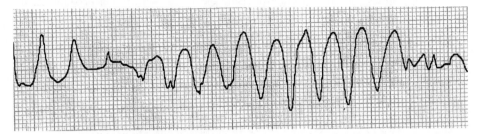

Figure 10.16 Torsades de pointes.

What is the QRS rate?	Greater than 120 bpm
Is the QRS rhythm regular?	No
What is the QRS duration?	Prolonged, greater than 0.12 s (three small squares)
Is there atrial activity?	Not discernable
Are there P waves before each QRS?	Not discernable
What is the PR interval?	Not discernable

Arrhythmia treatment

In very simple terms, the treatments for all arrhythmias fall under five headings.

- *Vagal manoeuvres.* A number of physical manoeuvres can increase para-sympathetic activity, which slows conduction through the AV node. These are used for supraventricular tachycardia and include carotid sinus massage and the Valsalva manoeuvre (forced expiration against a closed glottis). These techniques may also act as a diagnostic aid, for example to determine whether a narrow complex tachycardia is atrial flutter (Nolan et al., 2005).
- *Defibrillation.* A very short-duration electric current is passed through the heart, usually via electrodes placed on the chest wall. This causes simul-taneous depolarisation of most of the myocardium, with the hope that in the repolarisation phase which follows, normal conduction will occur. This is used to treat VF and pulseless VT. Cardioversion is an elective or semi-elective procedure used to terminate other arrhythmias. In this procedure, the patient is anaesthetised and the defibrillator is set (synchronised) to deliver the shock on the R wave of the patient's ECG. This reduces the risk of provoking VF by firing on the T wave. In recent years, automated implantable cardioverter devices (ICDs) have been increasingly used in patients at risk of sudden arrhythmic deaths.

- *Pacemakers.* These devices stimulate the myocardium, using short, intermittent pulses of current. The current can be applied transcutaneously using pads on the chest wall, through a transvenous electrode that has its tip on the endocardium or using electrodes on the epicardium. So, for example, if a patient has complete heart block, with a slow ventricular rate, the pacemaker current can be set to pulse at 70 times per minute, directly stimulating ventricular myocardium to depolarise at that rate. Implantable pacemakers have been used since the late 1950s (Zipes and Wellens, 2000) and have become highly sophisticated, programmable devices, used to treat tachyarrhythmias as well as bradycardias.
- *Drug therapy.* As all anti-arrhythmic drugs work by inhibiting the ion channels or ion pumps that generate the action potential, they may also cause arrhythmias, hypotension and heart failure (also discussed in Chapter 8). They can be divided into five categories (ESC, 1991).
  - Class I – Na^+ channel blockers. Class 1A drugs prolong the action potential (e.g. mexilitine), useful for the treatment of ventricular arrhythmias and recurrent atrial fibrillation. Class 1B drugs (e.g. lignocaine) shorten the action potential. Class 1C drugs (e.g. flecainide) have no effect on the action potential, and are used in the treatment of recurrent tachyarrhythmias and paroxysmal atrial fibrillation.
  - Class II – beta-blockers (e.g. atenolol). Used to decrease mortality in post-myocardial infarction patients, and can prevent the recurrence of tachyarrhythmias. Beta-blockers decrease heart rate by slowing the force of contraction by decreasing the sensitivity of the cardiac cells that act as receptors to adrenaline.
  - Class III – K^+ channel blockers (e.g. amiodarone). Used in patients with Wolff–Parkinson–White syndrome, ventricular tachycardia and atrial flutter and fibrillation. These drugs bind to and block the potassium channels that are responsible for phase 3 of the action potential (Figure 10.2), repolarisation. This leads to an increased action potential duration and hence a prolonged QT interval on the ECG.
  - Class IV – Ca^{2+} channel blockers (e.g. verapamil). Used to help prevent recurrence of paroxysmal supraventricular tachycardia. Also used to reduce the ventricular rate in patients with atrial fibrillation. These drugs block the calcium channel during the plateau phase (*see* Figure 10.2) of the action potential and thus slow the conduction of the heart hopefully resulting in a decreased heart rate.
  - Class V – other anti arrhythmic drugs (e.g. adenosine). Used to treat supraventricular tachycardia. Since the inception of the Vaughan-Williams drug classification scale, many drugs developed do not fit within the classes previously discussed and therefore Class V has been introduced. They all work slightly differently, and the reader is encouraged to look up each individual drug to assess how it works and its effects on the action potential.
- *Electrical ablation of abnormal pathways.* Abnormal areas of conduction are accurately located and destroyed with radiofrequency-generated heat

or laser probes (rarely cold is used externally). This ends the disturbance in the electrical circuit and restores normal conduction. If other methods, lifestyle and drug therapy have not worked, cardiac ablation is a successful next treatment in more than 90% of cases (Paradis et al., 2007).

Peri-arrest arrhythmias

In the peri-arrest patient, bradyarrhythmias and tachyarrhythmias may wholly or partially contribute to reduced cardiac output, and guidelines have been described for the emergency management of these (Nolan et al., 2005). These guidelines are revised regularly, the current guidance being available on the Resuscitation Council (UK) website.

These patients should be given high concentration oxygen and a venous cannula should be inserted.

Bradycardias

A rapid assessment is made of the patient to decide whether they have adverse signs or a risk of asystole. Adverse signs include heart failure, heart rate less than 40, hypotension and bradycardia with ventricular arrhythmias. Risk factors for asystole include previous asystole, Mobitz type 2 second degree heart block, complete heart block with a QRS duration greater than 0.12 s and pauses in ventricular activity for longer than 3 s. Treatment for both groups will include giving atropine 500 µg boluses, up to a maximum of 3 mg. If this does not increase the heart rate or improve symptoms, cardiology advice should be sought and transcutaneous or transvenous pacing or an isoprenaline infusion should be commenced.

Tachycardias

Again, a rapid assessment is made of the patient to decide whether they are stable or unstable. Signs of instability include chest pain, reduced level of consciousness, hypotension or heart failure. Unstable patients are treated with DC cardioversion. Stable patients are treated with drugs, for example amiodarone for AF or VT, adenosine for SVT and magnesium for torsade. For all of these patients, cardiology advice should be sought.

Cardiac arrest rhythms

Cardiac arrhythmias can be sporadic and variable within medical cardiac emergencies. Interpretation of such arrhythmias, particularly those of cardiac arrest, plays an important role within the instigation of early, appropriate medical management. Early definitive treatment is essential to optimise chances of survival. Within this section the arrhythmias of ventricular

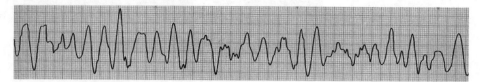

Figure 10.17 Ventricular fibrillation (VF).

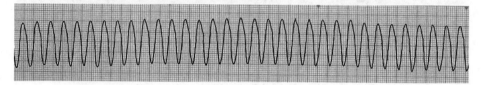

Figure 10.18 Ventricular tachycardia (VT) (as described on page 146).

tachycardia (VT), ventricular fibrillation (VF), asystole and electromechanical dissociation (EMD) will be discussed, within the paradigms of shockable and non-shockable rhythms (Resuscitation Council, 2010).

Shockable rhythms (VF/VT)

In adults, the commonest rhythm at the time of cardiac arrest is VF (Figure 10.17), which may be preceded by a period of VT (Figures 10.15, 10.16 and 10.18), by a bradyarrhythmia, or less commonly, supraventricular tachycardia (SVT).

Ventricular fibrillation

There is chaotic, uncoordinated ventricular depolarisation. The synchronous contraction of the ventricles is lost, with groups of cells at different stages of depolarisation and repolarisation. In the exposed heart the ventricles appear to quiver. This is a rhythm of cardiac arrest: the pumping action of the ventricles ceases and death will ensue within minutes unless a defibrillatory shock is applied.

Treatment of shockable rhythms (VF/VT)

Having confirmed cardiac arrest, summon help (including a request for a defibrillator) and start CPR, beginning with chest compressions, with a compression: ventilation ratio of 30:2. As soon as the defibrillator arrives apply self-adhesive pads or paddles to the chest to diagnose the rhythm. If VF/VT is confirmed, follow the treatment steps below.

- Attempt defibrillation. Give one shock of 150/200 J biphasic (360 J monophasic), the exact joules to be given will be determined by your trust guidelines – ensure that you are familiar with these.
- Immediately resume uninterrupted chest compressions (30:2) without reassessing the rhythm or feeling for a pulse. It is important throughout to

reduce the pre-shock pause by ensuring chest compressions are conti-
nued without interruptions.
- Continue CPR for 2 min, then pause briefly to check the monitor.
  - If VF/VT persists:
    - give a further (second) shock of 150–360 J biphasic (360 J
      monophasic)
    - resume CPR immediately and continue for 2 min
    - pause briefly to check the monitor
    - If VF/VT persists give a (third) shock of 150–360 J biphasic (360 J
      monophasic)
    - resume CPR immediately and continue for 2 min. Once CPR has been
      recommenced, give adrenaline 1 mg IV and amiodorone 300 mg IV.
    - pause briefly to check the monitor
    - if VF/VT persists give a (fourth) shock of 150–360 J biphasic (360 J
      monophasic)
    - resume CPR immediately and continue for 2 min
    - give adrenaline 1 mg IV after alternate shocks (i.e. approximately
      every 3–5 min)
    - give further shocks after each 2 min period of CPR and after confirm-
      ing that VF/VT persists.
  - If organised electrical activity compatible with a cardiac output is seen,
    check for a pulse:
    - if a pulse is present, start post-resuscitation care
    - if no pulse is present, continue CPR and switch to the non-shockable
      algorithm.
  - If asystole is seen, continue CPR and switch to the non-shockable
    algorithm.

Non-shockable rhythms (PEA and asystole)

Pulseless electrical activity (PEA)
PEA is defined as organised cardiac electrical activity in the absence of any
palpable pulses – it can be any rhythm that one would normally expect to
have an associated cardiac output. These patients often have some mechanical myocardial contractions but they are too weak to produce a detectable
pulse or blood pressure. PEA may be caused by reversible conditions that
can be treated. Survival following cardiac arrest with asystole or PEA is unlikely
unless a reversible cause can be found and treated quickly and effectively.

Asystole (Figure 10.19)
Often referred to as a flat line, it is very rarely a flat line, rather, an undulat-
ing base line is seen. There is no electrical activity and hence no contraction
of the heart muscle and no blood flow.

Treatment for PEA/asystole
- Start CPR 30:2.
- Give adrenaline 1 mg IV/IO as soon as access is achieved.

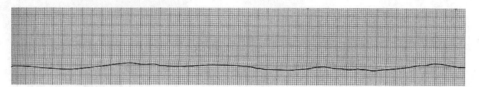

Figure 10.19 Asystole.

- Continue CPR 30:2 until the airway is secured - then continue chest compressions without pausing during ventilation.
- Recheck the rhythm after 2 min
    - If organised electrical activity is seen, check for a pulse and/or signs of life:
        - if a pulse andor signs of life are present, start post-resuscitation care
        - if no pulse and/or no signs of life are present (PEA):
            - continue CPR
            - recheck the rhythm after 2 min and proceed accordingly
            - give further adrenaline 1 mg IV/IO every 3-5 min (alternate loops).
    - If VF/VT at rhythm check, change to shockable side of algorithm.
    - If asystole or an agonal rhythm seen at rhythm check:
        - continue CPR
        - recheck the rhythm after 2 min and proceed accordingly
        - give adrenaline 1 mg IV/IO every 3-5 min (alternate loops).

Treatment for asystole and slow PEA (rate <60 min)

- Start CPR 30:2.
- Check that the leads are attached correctly without stopping CPR.
- Give adrenaline 1 mg IV as soon as IV access is achieved.
- Continue CPR 30:2 until the airway is secured - then continue chest compressions without pausing during ventilation.
- Recheck the rhythm after 2 min and proceed accordingly.
- If VF/VT recurs, change to the shockable rhythm algorithm.
- Give adrenaline 1 mg IV every 3-5 min (alternate loops).

Asystole

Whenever a diagnosis of asystole is made, check the ECG carefully for the presence of P waves, because in this situation ventricular standstill may be treated effectively by cardiac pacing. Attempts to pace true asystole are unlikely to be successful (Resuscitation Council, 2010). Treatment options are summarised in the ALS algorithm (Figure 10.20).

Reversible causes

In recent years, the management of cardiac arrest has moved from simply treating the cardiac arrest to attempting to treat its cause, potential causes

Adult Advanced Life Support

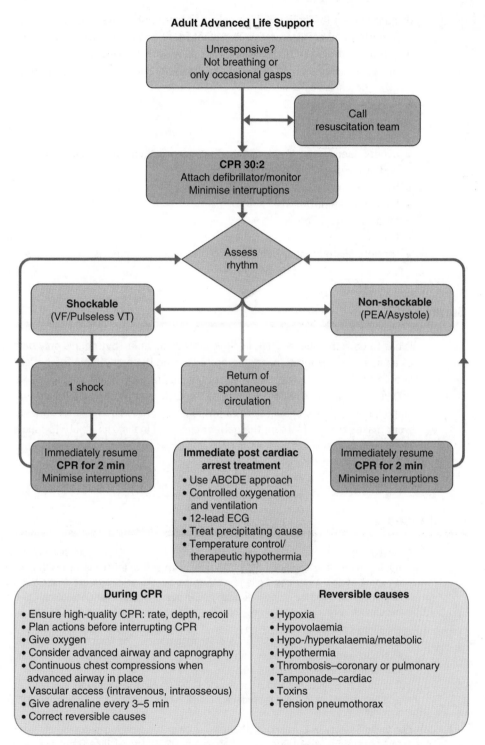

Figure 10.20 Resuscitation Council (2010) adult advanced life support algorithm. Reproduced with permission of Resuscitation Council (UK).

or aggravating factors for which specific treatment exists must be considered during any cardiac arrest. The eight more common causes have been grouped, according to their initial letter, as Hs and Ts. This is to make them easier to remember in an emergency (Resuscitation Council, 2010) (Figure 10.20). They are:

- hypoxia
- hypovolaemia
- hyperkalaemia, hypokalaemia, hypoglycaemia, hypocalcaemia, acidaemia and other metabolic disorders
- hypothermia
- tension pneumothorax
- cardiac-tamponade
- toxins
- thrombosis (pulmonary embolism or coronary thrombosis).

Summary

It has to be remembered that, in clinical practice, an arrhythmia is only part of a patient's presentation, and before analysing the arrhythmia the patient should be assessed. Applying a systematic approach when looking at an arrhythmia, finding the components of the ECG complex and their relationship can simplify its description. Knowledge of how arrhythmia treatments work makes their effects on the patient clearer. Finally, the ability to follow clear, scientifically derived guides for management of cardiac arrest optimises the patient's chances of survival.

References

Blomstrom-Lindqvist C, Scheinmann MM, Aliot EM *et al*. (2003) ACC/AHA/ESC guidelines for the management of patients with supraventricular arrhythmias: a report of the American College of Cardiology/ American Heart Association task force on practice guidelines and the European Society for Cardiology committee on practice guidelines 2003. *Journal of the American College of Cardiology* **42**(8): 1493–531.

Cobbe SM and Rankin AC (1993) Cardiac arrhythmias. In: Warrell DA, Cox TM, Firth JD and Benz EJ (eds) The Oxford Textbook of Medicine (4e). Oxford University Press, Oxford, pp. 2981–96.

Dobrzynski H, Boyett MR and Anderson RH (2007) New insights into pacemaker activity. Promoting understanding of sick sinus syndrome. *Circulation* **115**: 1921–32.

European Society of Cardiology: the task force of the working group on arrhythmias of the European Society of Cardiology (1991) The Sicilian Gambit. A new approach to the classification of antiarrhythmic drugs based on their actions on arrhythmogenic mechanisms. *Circulation* **84**: 1831–51.

Fuster V, Ryden LE, Cannom DS *et al*. (2006) ACC/AHA/ESC 2006 guidelines for the management of atrial fibrillation: a report of the American College of Cardiology/American Heart Association task force on practice guidelines and the European Society for Cardiology committee on practice guidelines. *Europace* **8**: 651-745.

Grant AO and Durrani S (2007) Mechanisms of cardiac arrhythmias. In: Topol EJ (ed.) Textbook of Cardiovascular Medicine (3e). Philadelphia, Lippincott Williams and Wilkins.

Hoffman BF and Rosen MR (1981) Cellular mechanisms for cardiac arrhythmias. *Circulation Research* **49**(1): 1-15.

Narula OS and Samet P (1970) Wenkebach and Mobitz type II A-V block due to block within the His bundle and bundle branches. *Circulation* **41**: 947-65.

Nolan JP, Deakin CD, Soar J, Bottiger BW and Smith G (2005) European Resuscitation Council guidelines for resuscitation 2005. Section 4. Adult advanced life support. *Resuscitation* **67**(S1): S39-S86.

Paradis NA, Halperin HR, Kern KB, Wenzel V and Chamberlain DA (2007) Cardiac Arrest. The Science and Practice of Resuscitation Medicine (2e). Cambridge, Cambridge University Press.

Resuscitation Council UK (2010) Advanced Life Support Provider Manual (6e). London, Resuscitation Council UK.

Samie FH and Jose J (2001) Mechanisms underlying ventricular tachycardia and its transition to ventricular fibrillation in the structurally normal heart. *Cardiovascular Research* **50**: 242-50.

Schamroth L (1990) Electrocardiography, An Introduction. Oxford, Blackwell Scientific Publications.

Wolbrette DL and Nacarelli GV (2007) Bradycardias: sinus node dysfunction and atrioventricular conduction disturbances. In: Topol EJ (ed.) Textbook of Cardiovascular Medicine (3e). Philadelphia, Lippincott Williams and Wilkins.

Zipes DP and Wellens HJJ (2000) What have we learned about cardiac arrhythmias? *Circulation* **102**: IV52-IV57.

Web resources

European Resuscitation Council, www.erc.edu
European Society for cardiology, www.escardio.org
Resuscitation Council (UK), www.resus.org.uk
Wikipedia (2009), www.wikipedia.org/wiki/Heartbeat

Chapter 11
Emergency Cardiac Care
Melanie Humphreys and Lisa Cooper

Introduction

Cardiovascular emergencies are life-threatening disorders that must be assessed and diagnosed quickly to avoid a delay in treatment and to minimise morbidity and mortality – they may be sudden events or may be preceded by a noticeable deterioration in the patient's condition. Activity, levels of anxiety, speed of onset and previous experience may influence the patient's perception of the significance of their illness and its severity. Sudden cardiac emergencies are particularly distressing and frightening, not only for patients but also for the carers (Humphreys, 2009).

Virtually every pathological process affecting the heart can lead to a critical cardiac event and, commonly, sudden death, therefore a good understanding of emergency cardiac events and their immediate management is essential for reducing this risk. Through a structured approach of assessment, initiating investigations, treatment and delivering appropriate care, potential life-threatening cardiac events can be identified, alerting medical staff immediately to these situations and ensuring the most appropriate evidence-based treatment strategies are adopted. This chapter discusses the assessment of the deteriorating patient and care of patients with a range of emergency cardiovascular events; Chapter 10 has examined arrhythmias and resuscitation.

Nursing the Cardiac Patient, First Edition. Edited by Melanie Humphreys.
© 2011 Blackwell Publishing Ltd. Published 2011 by Blackwell Publishing Ltd.

> ## Learning outcomes
>
> The aim of this chapter is to understand the treatment and management of the deteriorating patient and common cardiac emergencies. At the end of this chapter the reader will be able to:
>
> - describe the systematic approach to assessment of the deteriorating patient and how to apply this to a MEWS process
> - describe the priorities of nursing care for patients with acute cardiac emergencies
> - describe the causes, presentation and management of a range of acute cardiac events and electrolyte disorders.

Cardiac emergencies in perspective

Over the past few years outreach teams have been set up to facilitate the appropriate care of deteriorating patients and provide support for staff who are looking after them – often modified early warning scores (MEWS; NCEPOD, 2005) are used to instigate the alert of such teams (Resuscitation Council, 2010). It is becoming more common that acutely ill patients are being cared for on general wards, which can place them at high risk. Seventy-nine percent of patients, who experience in-hospital cardiac arrest display basic signs of physiological deterioration before they collapse. Although cardiac events are common everyday occurrences, it is startling to find that some studies suggest that many critically ill patients have cardiac arrest because of inadequate initial assessment and subsequent non-recognition of patient deterioration (Resuscitation Council, 2010). As a result of these findings, guidelines are now aimed at improving detection of deteriorating patients and the prevention of subsequent cardiac arrest (NICE, 2007; NPSA, 2007).

The ALERT (Acute Life Threatening Events Recognition and Treatment) course was developed by Portsmouth University and is now provided nationally (Smith, 2003). The aim of this course is to provide education to a safe standard of basic competencies in caring for acutely ill patients. SBAR – Situation, Background, Assessment and Recommendations – was constructed to aid nurses in their communication of vital information to their medical and nursing colleagues (Haig et al., 2006). Fundamentally, these approaches to acute care enable practitioners to assess patients correctly and to convey their findings to their colleagues.

Early warning scoring systems

The early warning score (EWS) was developed as a scoring system to be used at ward level; physiological parameters such as blood pressure, pulse rate,

	Points						
	3	2	1	0	1	2	3
Systolic BP	<70	71–80	81–100	101–199		≥200	
Pulse		<40	41–50	51–100	101–110	111–129	>130
Respiratory		<9		9–14	15–20	21–29	>30
Temperature		<35		35–38.4		>38.5	
Neurological score (AVPU)			New agitation or confusion	Alert	Reacting to Voice	Reacting to Pain	Completely Unresponsive
Urine output	<10 ml/h	<20 ml/h					

Figure 11.1 An example of a modified early warning score (MEWS) system.

respiratory rate, AVPU score (is the patient Alert, responding to Voice, Responding to Pain or Unconscious; *see* Figure 11.1), temperature and urine output are used to identify the early deterioration of the patient. Deviations from the "normal" ranges are then scored and a total is calculated. The total score then guides the clinical staff to further actions, i.e. alerting the critical care outreach team (CCOT).

In the years since the publication of comprehensive critical care (DH, 2000), CCOTs have developed across most acute hospitals in England. However, this has not happened in a uniform manner. Services still vary in the hours that they are available, the amount of dedicated medical input, the number and position of nursing staff involved, and the overall approach of the team (Deacon, 2009).

Multiprofessional CCOTs by their very nature have an advantage when communicating with different disciplines across hospital environments. The majority of CCOTs that have shown measurable benefits have been multiprofessional (Cutler and Robson, 2006). There is variety in the amount of medical input into CCOTs and most services are nurse led, Gao *et al.*, (2007) reported that 71.1% of services had no medical input at all.

In recent clinical guidance relating to the acutely ill hospital patient, the National Institute for Health and Clinical Excellence (NICE, 2007) reviewed available evidence relating to track-and-trigger systems being used internationally. While the evidence was able to suggest some pros and cons of different systems, it was felt there wasn't sufficient evidence to recommend one particular system over another. One thing that is clear is the recommendation that *all* adult patients in acute hospital settings should be monitored with a track-and-trigger system, but the choice of which particular system to use should be decided at a local level.

The MEWS is an example of an aggregate scoring track-and-trigger system and is used widely in the UK (Figure 11.1). A MEWS score of 2 in *any* single category indicates the need for close and frequent observation of the patient. A MEWS score of 4 and/or an increase of 2 or more indicates that the patient is potentially unwell and means that urgent medical attention is required. While it has been established that physiological abnormality is associated with adverse outcome, within a recent Cochrane review it was stated that the use of early warning scores or outreach calling criteria in the practice setting needs to be evaluated. This would provide an understanding of the factors associated with poor documentation of EWS charts and the reluctance of ward staff to use the calling criteria (McGaughey, 2009).

Assessing the emergency cardiac patient

For all patients who present with a possible cardiac emergency, the initial nursing assessment should be focused, specific and efficiently undertaken. It follows the same approach that can be used for the assessment of all groups of patients.

A – Airway

- Ensure the patient's airway is patent, i.e. is the patient talking to you?
- Administer oxygen therapy as indicated via the appropriate oxygen delivery device at 15 l high flow oxygen.

B – Breathing

- Look at the patient – are they pale or are there any signs of cyanosis?
- What is their respiratory rate?
- What is their respiratory effort like? Are they using any accessory muscles?
- Are they speaking full sentences or do they have to keep stopping to take a breath?

C – Circulation

- Pulses – are they all present? Are they equal on both sides?
- What is the rate? What is the volume like? Are there any particular characteristics? i.e. regular/irregular?
- Blood pressure – what is it? Is it equal on both sides?
- Electrocardiogram (ECG) – three-lead monitor should be attached and 12-lead ECG undertaken as soon as possible, dependent on the patient's condition, to assess for abnormalities.
- Intravenous (IV) access should be gained and bloods taken – appropriate for their presenting problem and local guidelines.

- IV analgesia should also be given at this point if indicated.
- Care should be taken with opioid analgesia – see specific sections.

D – Disability

- How is the patient responding?
- Use the AVPU scale to assess the patient – are they alert (A), responsive to voice (V), responsive to pain (P) or are they unresponsive (U)?
- Pupils – are they equal and reactive to light?

E – Exposure

- Prepare the patient for full examination while keeping them warm and preserving their dignity.

Additional information

While undertaking the above assessment, there is information that is needed to be gained from the patient about themselves and their presenting complaint. This further information can be remembered using the mnemonic SAMPLE.

S – Signs and **S**ymptoms

- What were the signs and symptoms that led to concern for the patient/ practitioner?
- Signs – things you can see or hear.
- Symptoms – things the patient reports.

A – Allergies

- Are they allergic to any medications?
- Are they allergic to any other product you may use on them, i.e. Elastoplast, latex?

M – Medication

- What medications do they normally take?
- What dose do they normally take?
- Have they taken it today as normal?
- Do any of their medications have cardiac side effects?
- Are they on any new medications that maybe reacting with others?

P – Past medical history

- Is there any relevant history?
- Are they known to have any cardiac problems?
- Have they got any respiratory problems?

L - Last eaten

- The time of their last drink or food – can be relevant if they require any sedation or anaesthetic.

E - Events

- Events of this episode.
- What happened?
- When did it happen?
- What were they doing when it happened?
- Were there any witnesses to the event?
- Have they had similar episodes before?
- If so, what happened then?
- What was the outcome/diagnosis?

By using this systematic assessment, patients with possible cardiac emergencies can be quickly and thoroughly assessed. The level of intervention will vary depending on the nurse's skill, e.g. does the nurse have the ability to insert an IV cannula, and are they a nurse prescriber.

Reassurance also plays a large part in the management of these patients. Patients with cardiac emergencies tend to be frightened and this in turn puts a greater strain on their cardiac system. Therefore they need reassurance, which also includes the need to be treated in a calm environment by a team of staff who have a calm demeanour.

Acute heart failure

Heart failure is a major cause of morbidity and mortality in the Western world and the incidence of heart failure is increasing because of the ageing population.

Heart failure is an abnormality of cardiac structure or function that reduces the heart's ability to eject blood (systolic dysfunction) or fill with blood (diastolic dysfunction). Acute heart failure is a sudden reduction in cardiac performance, resulting in acute pulmonary oedema. Clinical and radiographic assessment of these patients provides a guide to the severity and prognosis (Millane *et al.*, 2000). There is an accumulation of fluid within the alveolar spaces which leads to the lungs becoming stiff, and subsequently gaseous exchange is impaired leading to worsening hypoxaemia and hypercapnia, which is life threatening. The major effects of heart failure are reduced organ perfusion, arrhythmias and vasoconstriction, which in turn cause their own problems (Souhami and Moxham, 2002).

Causes

Pulmonary oedema is an abnormal amount of interstitial fluid in the interstitial spaces and alveoli. The oedema may arise from increased pulmonary capillary permeability (pulmonary origin) or from an increase in pulmonary capillary pressure (cardiac origin) and heart failure. As the heart becomes less effective, more blood remains in the ventricles at the end of each cardiac cycle and therefore the end-diastolic volume (pre-load) increases. If the left ventricle is the first to fail, it becomes unable to pump out all of the blood it receives so it backs up in the lungs, causing increased pulmonary pressure. Whereas if the right ventricle fails first, the blood backs up systemically, i.e. pedal oedema (Tortora and Derrickson, 2008).

Heart failure may occur due to a combination of factors such as:

- pneumonia (common in elderly patients)
- hypoxia
- cardiac ischaemia
- sepsis
- renal failure.

The main differential diagnosis that can be mistakenly diagnosed as heart failure is acute exacerbation of chronic obstructive pulmonary disease (COPD) as it is often difficult to distinguish between the two. Therefore care is required when taking the patient's history, including past medical history. It is imperative that the diagnosis of heart failure is accompanied by an urgent attempt to establish its cause, as timely intervention may greatly improve the prognosis in selected cases. Severe acute heart failure is a medical emergency, and effective management requires an assessment of the underlying cause, improvement of the haemodynamic status, relief of pulmonary congestion and improved tissue oxygenation. In patients with acute heart failure, an underlying infection is common (Sprigings and Chambers, 2001).

Contributing factors

- Genetic family history of heart failure.
- Ischaemic heart disease/myocardial infarction (coronary artery disease) leading to reduced cardiac function.
- Thyrotoxicosis (hyperthyroidism).
- Arrhythmias.
- Hypertension – long-term increases the afterload of the heart.
- Cardiac fibrosis.
- Coarctation of the aorta.
- Aortic stenosis/regurgitation.
- Mitral regurgitation.
- Pulmonary stenosis/pulmonary hypertension/pulmonary embolism.
- Mitral valve disease.

Presentation

These patients are often acutely unwell and extremely frightened and agitated, can be mildly aggressive and do not like oxygen masks as they feel they restrict their breathing even more.

Their presentation includes the following.

- Acute shortness of breath which is usually the first symptom and may be the reason the patient presents themselves to a practitioner.
- Often the patient may collapse.
- Pallor and/or cyanosis which is often a late sign.
- Unable to speak full sentences.
- Agitation.
- Diaphoresis.
- Raised jugular venous pressure (JVP).
- Low volume pulse.
- Ankle/pedal oedema.
- Muffled heart sounds on auscultation.
- Feeble pulse.
- Often hypertension.

Other associated features which may reflect underlying cause include the following.

- Chest pain may be present.
- Palpitations may also be present.
- Dyspnoea on exertion, which is an early sign and may be present for some weeks before the patient seeks advice.
- Orthopnoea may also have been present for some weeks before.

Priorities of assessment

For this group of patients the priorities initially are as follows.

- Assess the patient following the ABCDE approach.
- Administer oxygen therapy as indicated via the appropriate oxygen delivery device; sit the patient in an upright position.
- Establish oxygen saturation monitoring using a pulse oximeter. Be aware that SpO_2 may not give accurate reading due to peripheral shutdown.
- Ensure patient has a wide-bore IV cannula in place (e.g. 14 gauge).
- Establish continuous ECG monitoring; and undertake a 12-lead ECG.
- Closely monitor the patient's vital signs with frequent reassessments – deterioration may be rapid; include blood pressure, temperature, pulse and respiratory rate. Close observation and frequent reassessment are required in the early hours of treatment.

- Prepare for transfer to high-dependency care area. Patients with acute severe heart failure, or refractory symptoms, should be monitored in a high-dependency unit.
- Urinary catheterisation facilitates accurate assessment of fluid balance, maintenance of >30 ml/h.
- Arterial blood gases monitoring; this provide valuable information regarding oxygenation and acid-base balance.
- Reassurance is vital with this group of patients as they will be extremely frightened and distressed.

Monitor vital signs with frequent reassessment (blood pressure, pulse, respiration rate, ECG and urine output). An arterial line can be inserted for ease of obtaining arterial blood gases and also to monitor BP more accurately. In severe cases the patient may require continuous positive airway pressure ventilation (CPAP) to assist their breathing. Remember a "normal" blood pressure can be maintained by vasoconstriction and does not indicate adequate organ perfusion (Sprigings and Chambers, 2001).

The aims of treatment are to:

- reduce the symptoms of dyspnoea (most important)
- reduce cardiac filling pressures
- reduce excess intravascular volume
- reduce vascular resistance
- increase cardiac output.

Treatment priorities

- Glyceryl trinitrate (GTN) infusion commencing at 0.6 mg/h dependent on the patient's blood pressure, i.e. systolic above 100 mm Hg – reduces preload and afterload and reduces ischaemia.
- Morphine titrated to patient's level of consciousness, 5–10 mg IV, accompanied by an anti-emetic, e.g. metochlopramide 10 mg IV – reduces anxiety and preload (venodilation), and reduces myocardial oxygen demand but is also a respiratory suppressant, so caution is required.
- Furosemide 40–80 mg IV – induces venodilation and dieresis.
- Blood tests – urea and electrolytes (U&Es) to ascertain renal function, full blood count (FBC) to ascertain if anaemia is present.
- Chest X-ray – confirms diagnosis and also to ascertain if infection or effusion is present (Figure 11.2).
- May require inotropic support in later stages should hypotension occur to maintain blood pressure, i.e. dobutamine 5 µg/kg/min – increases myocardial contractility.

Pericarditis

The pericardium is a fibrous sac that provides support for the heart (Figure 11.3). Similar to the pleura, the pericardium may be affected by inflammation,

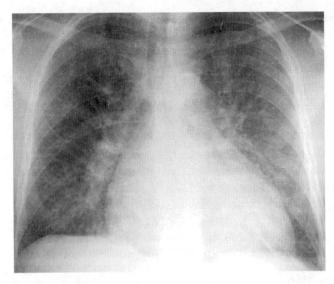

Figure 11.2   Chest X-ray showing acute heart failure.

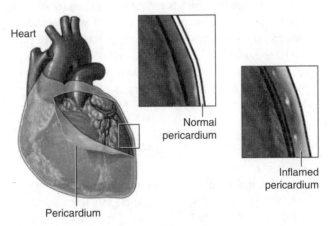

Heart

Normal
pericardium

Inflamed
pericardium

Pericardium

Figure 11.3   The pericardium. Reproduced with permission from John Wiley
& Sons.

infiltration by neoplasms, calcification and also fluid accumulation (Souhami
and Moxham, 2002).

Pericarditis is a common cardiovascular condition and is due to an inflammation of the pericardium causing a painful rubbing together of the parietal
and visceral pericardial layers. Pericarditis is further classified according to
the composition of the inflammatory exudate: serous, purulent, fibrinous and
haemorrhagic types are distinguished (Kumar and Clark, 2000). Acute pericarditis is more common than chronic pericarditis, and occurs most commonly due to viral infection or idiopathic causes. A diagnosis of acute
pericarditis is challenging due to the clinical presentation, which can be a
confusing picture.

Causes

- Idiopathic.
- Infection – viral, bacterial, TB.
  - Viral pericarditis – 25% can recur; this may be due to an auto-immune disorder and should be investigated (Sohami and Moxham, 2002).
- Dressler's syndrome – auto-immune disorder that occurs post-cardiac surgery or MI.
- Malignancy – carcinoma of lung and breast are the most common.
- Auto-immune disorders such as systemic lupus erythematosus (SLE) and rheumatoid arthritis (RA).
- Hypothyroidism.
- Trauma to the heart resulting in infection or inflammation.
- Radiotherapy.
- Acute renal failure

Presentation

These patients typically present with positional central chest pain, often pleuritic in nature, which is relieved by sitting forward and worse when lying down. However, the pain can also present as a dull radiating chest discomfort that can mimic myocardial ischaemia. Radiation of the pain to the edge of the trapezius is a very common specific sign of pericardial inflammation due to irritation of the phrenic nerve, which can sometimes be relieved by leaning forward (McConachie and Roberts, 2000).

Their presentation includes the following.

- The patient is often breathless.
- Cough with or without fever may also be present.
- Anxiety.
- ECG changes – initially there may be "saddle-shaped" ST segment elevation making it difficult to distinguish from acute MI; this is present in 60–70% of pericarditic patients (Figure 11.4) (Wyatt et al., 1998). This may progress after the initial few days into T wave inversion (Nolan et al., 1998).
- Troponin I levels may be raised in up to a third of pericarditic patients, which can lead to misdiagnosis of MI.
- Pericardial effusion is common in up to 60% of cases but only 10% of these are severe and it is more common in acute rather than chronic pericarditis (Davey, 2006).
- Friction rub on chest auscultation may also be heard in the majority of cases; it is normally along the lower left sternal border and is increased on leaning forward. However, it may not be present initially (Wyatt et al., 1998).
- If the chronic pericarditis is due to TB or post-chemotherapy and it becomes restrictive, then progressive exertional dyspnoea, peripheral oedema and also ascites may be present (Davey, 2006).

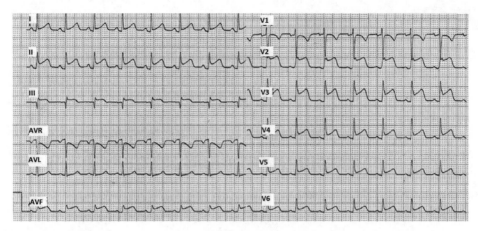

Figure 11.4 12-lead ECG showing saddle-shaped ST segments V₂–V₆.

Treatment priorities

This group of patients need to be nursed sitting in an upright position which is more comfortable for them.

- ABCDE, as in all patients.
- Monitor blood pressure, pulse, respiration rate, SpO₂, ECG – 3- and 12-lead.
- Blood tests – U&Es, FBC, C-reactive protein (CRP) and ESR for signs of infection and inflammation, and blood cultures where appropriate.
- Chest X-ray for heart size, pulmonary oedema, effusion and infection.
- Computed tomography (CT) and/or echocardiogram can be useful in diagnosis if they are available.
- Analgesia and non-steroidal anti-inflammatory drugs (NSAIDs) if there are no contra-indications.
- Steroids to reduce the inflammation.
- Antibiotics if bacterial infection is suspected.
- If viral cause, supportive treatment and symptom relief.
- Symptoms usually subside in approximately two weeks.

If effusion is large enough, subsequent haemodynamic compromise will occur, which can lead to cardiac tamponade (Myerson *et al.*, 2010).

Should drainage of fluid be required (pericardiocentesis), fluid should be sent for Ziehl-Nielson staining to rule out TB (Myerson *et al.*, 2010).

Cardiac tamponade

The pericardial cavity is a potential space between the parietal and visceral layers of the pericardium. This cavity normally contains between 30 and

50 ml of serous fluid that acts as a lubricant as the heart contracts and relaxes. This volume can increase to 1 litre in some chronic conditions, such as progressive malignant pericardial effusion with compromising pericardium. If fluid builds up gradually, the pericardium can stretch to contain as much as 1l of fluid without affecting the heart (Porth, 1994). However, if it accumulates rapidly, even an increase of as little as 50 ml can exert enough pressure on the heart to be life threatening (Humphreys, 2006, 2009). Indeed, cardiac tamponade is considered to be a life-threatening event.

Causes

The pericardium cannot stretch, so as the fluid accumulates within the pericardial sac, the diastolic pressure in each chamber rises so that filling the chambers is impaired (Thompson, 2005; Lilly, 1998).

The increase of systemic venous pressure results in signs of right-sided heart failure: distension of the jugular veins, oedema and hepatomegaly. Decreased atrial filling leads to inadequate ventricular filling, reduced cardiac output and potential circulatory collapse (Tortora and Derrickson, 2008). Pulsus paradoxus, in which arterial blood pressure during expiration exceeds arterial pressure during inspiration by more than 10 mm Hg, is a key indicator of cardiac tamponade. Normally, inspiration has little effect on cardiac flow or volume. In addition, reduced filling of the ventricles during diastole decreases blood availability for systolic stroke volume, and cardiac output declines. Failure to decompress the heart leads to inadequate perfusion of vital organs, shock and ultimately death (Resuscitation Council, 2010).

Other causes include:

* malignancy of the lung and breast
* acute MI which can lead to a free wall rupture as a complication of anti-coagulation (Sprigings and Chambers, 2001)
* Dressler's syndrome
* idiopathic pericarditis
* aortic dissection
* SLE.

Presentation

Cardiac tamponade should be suspected in any patient with known pericarditis, pericardial effusion or chest trauma who develops signs and symptoms of systemic vascular congestion and decreased cardiac output (Humphreys, 2006).

Key physical findings include:

* jugular venous distension
* systemic hypotension

- a small, quiet heart on physical examination (muffled heart sounds), due to the insulating effects of effusion (McCance and Huether, 1998).

Other signs include:

- sinus tachycardia and pulsus paradoxus
- dyspnoea and tachypnoea, which reflect pulmonary congestion, as well as decreased oxygen delivery to peripheral tissues.

Acute haemorrhage into the pericardium is also a result of left ventricular free wall rupture following MI, and frequently presents as chest pain, haemodynamic collapse and pulseless electrical activity (Connaughton, 2001). This occurs in between 1 and 4% of people post-MI and is usually rapidly fatal, in this instance the patient will present in cardiac arrest. During a cardiac arrest, cardiac tamponade is difficult to diagnose because the typical signs of distended neck veins and hypotension cannot be assessed. However, cardiac arrest after penetrating chest trauma should raise strong suspicions of tamponade (Dracup, 1995).

Differential diagnosis

Depending on the cause, cardiac tamponade can be misdiagnosed for the following disorders due to the similar presentations:

- aortic dissection
- pulmonary embolism
- acute severe asthma
- tension pneumothorax
- large pleural effusion.

Treatment priorities

The priorities initially are as follows.

- Assess the patient following the ABCDE approach.
- If the patient has altered consciousness level, his airway is at risk. Summon urgent medical help – this is a rapidly deteriorating life-threatening event.
- Administer oxygen therapy as indicated via the appropriate oxygen delivery device.
- Establish oxygen saturation monitoring using a pulse oximeter.
- Ensure the patient has a wide-bore IV cannula in place (e.g. 14 gauge).
- Establish continuous ECG monitoring; consider undertaking a 12-lead ECG. If tamponade has developed slowly over weeks or months, the ECG will share the characteristics of a pericardial effusion (Humphreys, 2006). In acute emergency situations, it is inappropriate to record a 12-lead ECG because immediate resuscitation and the removal of high-pressure pericardial fluid using pericardiocentesis or resuscitative thoracotomy are the

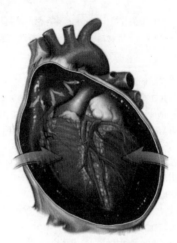

Figure 11.5 Cardiac tamponade. Reproduced with permission from John Wiley & Sons.

only measures that can reverse this life threatening condition (Humphreys, 2009; Resuscitation Council, 2010).
● Closely monitor the patient's vital signs with frequent reassessments – deterioration may be rapid; include blood pressure, temperature, pulse and respiratory rate.
● Prepare for immediate pericardiocentesis (undertaken by medical staff).

Cardiac tamponade is a life-threatening event; astute observations for the signs and symptoms of cardiac tamponade are critical to expedite treatment (Humphreys, 2006; Resuscitation Council, 2010) (Figure 11.5).

Electrolyte disorders

Electrolyte balance is maintained by oral, or in emergencies, IV intake of electrolyte-containing substances, and is regulated by hormones, generally with the kidneys flushing out excess levels. In humans, electrolyte homeostasis is regulated by hormones such as antidiuretic hormone, aldosterone and parathyroid hormone (Rose and Post, 2005). Serious electrolyte disturbances such as dehydration and over hydration may lead to cardiac and neurological complications and, unless they are rapidly resolved, will result in a medical emergency.

Excitability of myocardial tissue depends on the intracellular and extracellular concentrations of electrolytes, including potassium, sodium, magnesium and calcium, with myocardial excitability varying with changes in concentrations of these electrolytes (Clark, 2005). Electrolytes can either be intracellular or extracellular. Sodium is extracellular, whereas potassium, magnesium and calcium are intracellular. In addition, potassium chloride, magnesium sulphate and calcium chloride or gluconate are used effectively to manage cardiac arrhythmias. These drugs are used selectively in closely monitored situations as they are not without complications such as induced cardiac arrhythmias.

Potassium

Potassium levels are usually controlled by the uptake of potassium into the cells and excretion by the renal system (Souhami and Moxham, 2002). Potassium homeostasis is dependent on replacing daily losses in the urine and on adequate renal function. The kidney regulates serum potassium through active secretion of potassium into the distal tubule. Approximately 10% of hospitalised patients have hyperkalaemia, most often due to renal failure or hyperglycaemia, or medication that affect the levels of potassium (Kumar and Clark, 2000).

Potassium is regulated by the sodium-potassium ATP pump located on the plasma membrane of most cells. The kidney is the main route of excretion of potassium. Potassium is important for the repolarisation phase in muscles and neurons.

If potassium levels rise, an increase in aldosterone is triggered to prompt the kidneys to excrete more. If potassium levels fall, there is a reduction in aldosterone which in turn reduces the excretion by the kidneys (Clark, 2005).

Hyperkalaemia

Mild hyperkalaemia is classified as serum potassium greater than 6.0 mmol/l and severe hyperkalaemia is classified as serum potassium greater than 6.5 mmol/l (Davey, 2006).

Causes

Hyperkalaemia is a high concentration of potassium ions in the extracellular fluid and the main cause is renal failure due to the deficiency of potassium excretion (Davey, 2006).

High levels of potassium can be due to the following.

- Spurious – muscular activity either during physical activity or fist clenching during venepuncture, high platelet and/or leucocyte count.
- Transcellular shift – acidaemia in acute renal failure; hyperosmolarity, i.e. in diabetic ketoacidosis (DKA); beta-blocker use, i.e. propanolol; insulin deficiency, i.e. type I diabetes; and also in cell necrosis, i.e. after chemotherapy, which causes increased cellular release (Souhami and Moxham, 2002).
- Increased intake – increased potassium from specific foods/solutions, normal intake but with defect in excretion.
- Decreased excretion – mineral corticoid deficiency, i.e. Addison's disease; aldosterone deficiency; renin deficiency; NSAIDs use; severe renal failure.
- Cell death, i.e. burns, crush injury, which is due to potassium leaving the cells.

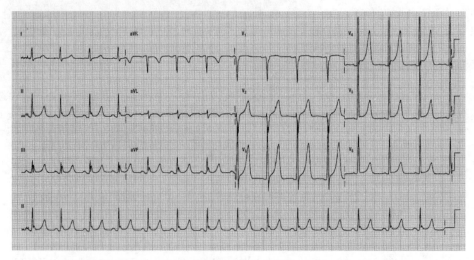

Figure 11.6 12-lead ECG with changes suggestive of hyperkalaemia.

Presentation

Presentation of hyperkalaemia is usually asymptomatic and is found on routine blood tests. However, patients can present with weakness, fatigue, palpitations, chest pain or occasionally collapse (Kumar and Clark, 2000). On assessment, the ECG will show peaked T waves and maybe a shortened QT interval, and also may show ST depression. If hyperkalaemia is severe then a widened QRS can lead to VT and VF (see Figure 11.6).

The ECG shows the following features:

- rapid and early R wave progression
- early transition zone V_2-V_3
- the T wave is tall, peaked and narrow in V_2-V_4 and more than two-thirds the height of the R wave – abnormal.

The diagnosis is sinus rhythm with T wave changes that are suggestive of hyperkalaemia. T wave changes do not need to be apparent in all leads – as evidenced here. The K^+ was 6.4 mmol/l in this patient.

Treatment priorities

- ABCDE as in all patients.
- Monitor ECG – 3- and 12-lead – to assess for changes.
- Monitor blood pressure, pulse, respiration rate and SpO_2.
- High levels of potassium can cause cardiac excitability, therefore calcium gluconate 10 ml/10% is given to protect the cell membranes from this effect.
- Insulin drives potassium into cells but must be given with glucose to avoid hypoglycaemia – 50 ml infusion of 10 units of Actrapid in 50% dextrose

over 30 min. Due to the action of insulin, blood glucose level must be closely monitored, especially if the patient is a diabetic.

- Nebulised salbutamol is highly effective, especially when combined with an insulin regime as it shifts potassium from the extracellular space into the intracellular space.
- Calcium or sodium resonium encourages the removal of potassium from the body via the gastrointestinal tract reverses membrane polarisation.

Hypokalaemia

Causes

Hypokalaemia is more common than hyperkalaemia and is the most common electrolyte disorder of hospitalised patients. It is most commonly due to diuretic therapy (Davey, 2006).

The most common cause of hypokalaemia is the prolonged use of diuretics, especially the thiazide group which encourage the excretion via the kidneys. The second most common cause, which is more common in the elderly age group, is gastrointestinal loss, i.e. diarrhoea and vomiting (Kumar and Clark, 2000). Other causes include the following.

- Excess IV fluids and inadequate intake, i.e. poor dietary intake.
- Alkalosis also leads to intracellular shift of potassium leading to hypokalaemia.
- Laxative abuse causes direct loss of potassium.
- Villous rectal adenoma causes enhanced potassium loss from tumour cells (Souhami and Moxham, 2002).

Presentation

Like hyperkalaemia, patients with hypokalaemia are usually asymptomatic and it is usually found on routine blood tests. However, patients may present with palpitations which can be due to a variety of arrhythmias, i.e. atrial tachycardia, supraventricular tachycardia and ventricular tachycardia, and ECG changes such as flattened T waves, ST depression or prolonged P-R interval (see Figure 11.7).

This chest lead shows massive U wave, ST depression and flat T waves; the K^+ was 1.6 mmol/l in this patient.

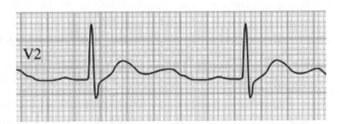

Figure 11.7 Single-lead ECG with changes suggestive of hypokalaemia.

Risks

Due to the nature of the arrhythmias, there is a risk that the patient may deteriorate into more serious arrhythmias such as torsades de point or ventricular fibrillation. Therefore close cardiac monitoring is essential in this group of patients.

If the patient is on digoxin, regular blood digoxin levels must be taken because of the risk of increased digoxin toxicity due to the increased binding of dogoaxin to cardiac cells, thereby potentiating its action.

Treatment priorities

- ABCDE as in all patients.
- Monitor ECG - 3- and 12-lead.
- Monitor blood pressure, pulse and respiration rate.
- If mild hypokalaemia is present then oral potassium may be sufficient. However. if the patient is symptomatic in any way, IV potassium will be necessary.

If the hypokalaemia is long standing it can lead to distal tubule damage (Davey, 2006).

Magnesium

Magnesium is stored in the bone matrix and is both extra- and intracellular. It is involved in the metabolism of carbohydrates and proteins. It is also important for neuromuscular activity and nerve impulse transmission, myocardial function and also in secretion of parathyroid hormone (PTH) (Clark, 2005).

Hypomagnesaemia

Fifty percent of the body's magnesium is in bones and the remaining 50% is in the tissues and organs. Magnesium helps maintain normal muscle and nerve function, supports the immune system and bone stability, and helps to maintain blood sugar levels.

Causes

The main causes of hypomagnesaemia include chronic alcoholism (malnutrition), gastrointestinal loss, impaired absorption (i.e. some cytotoxic treatments cause renal tubular damage which causes reduction in reabsorption) and increased excretion due to drugs, renal disease or diuretics (Souhami and Moxham, 2002).

Presentation

Once again these patients may be asymptomatic or may be acutely unwell. Early signs may include loss of appetite, nausea and vomiting, fatigue, weakness and then progress to tetany, palpitations, cramps and muscle contractions (Tortora and Derrickson, 2008). There is a high risk of serious cardiac complications (Souhami and Moxham, 2002) with hypomagnesaemia, i.e. atrial or ventricular tachycardia. In addition these patients may present with collapse and cardiogenic shock or heart failure.

Hypomagnesaemia can be linked to hypokalaemia and can also lead to hypocalcaemia.

Treatment priorities

- ABCDE as in all patients.
- Monitor ECG – 3- and 12-lead – to assess for ECG changes.
- Monitor blood pressure, pulse and respiration rate – usually in hypomagnesaemia, patients are tachycardic and hypotensive.
- Monitor neurological status for; weakness, tremors, tetany and parasthaesia.
- One has to remember that if magnesium levels are deranged then calcium levels will be also: if magnesium levels are high, then calcium levels will also be high; if magnesium levels are low then calcium levels will also be low.

Hypermagnesaemia

Hypermagnesaemia is classified as a serum magnesium of greater than 7.5 mmol/l.

Causes

Hypermagnesaemia is usually due to the intake being greater than the output, such as in renal failure or due to medications such as magnesium-containing antacids or laxatives.

Presentation

This group of patients usually present in a collapsed state complaining of lethargy and weakness, and they will display loss of deep tendon reflexes on examination. On further examination ECG changes will also be apparent, i.e. peaked T waves and a wide QRS. Therefore the patient may also complain of palpitations.

Risks

Increased magnesium levels depress cardiac conduction, which leads to bradycardia, complete heart block and asystole (Souhami and Moxham, 2002).

Treatment priorities

- ABCDE as in all patients.
- ECG – monitor 3- and 12-lead for ECG changes.
- Monitor blood pressure, pulse and respiration rate – hypermagnesaemia causes hypertension and bradycardia.

- Monitor neurological status for weakness and depressed deep tendon reflexes.
- The main aim of treatment is to treat the underlying cause, i.e. stop medications where appropriate, and to treat the symptoms where possible as they arise. In addition, calcium gluconate can be used to protect the cardiac cells from the excitability caused by the elevated magnesium.

Summary

As nurses expand their scope of practice they play an ever more important role in the management of patients who present with acute cardiac symptoms; virtually all pathological process affecting the heart can lead to a critical cardiac event and, commonly, sudden death. The nurse requires a good understanding of acute cardiac emergencies and electrolyte disturbances; understanding their immediate management is essential in reducing this risk. This chapter has examined the assessment and priorities of care for a range of acute cardiac events; nurses need an in-depth understanding of this important aspect of care in order to provide prompt, evidence-based treatments and respond quickly and appropriately to physiological compromise.

References

Clark R (2005) *Anatomy and Physiology: Understanding the Human Body*. London, Jones & Bartlett Publishers.

Connaughton M (2001) *Evidence-Based Coronary Care*. London, Churchill Livingston.

Cutler L and Robson W (2006) *Critical Care Outreach*. Chicester, John Wiley and Sons.

Davey P (2006) *Medicine at a Glance* (2e). Oxford, Blackwell Publishing.

Deacon K (2009) Critical care outreach service. In: Jevon P, Humphreys M and Ewens B (eds) (2009) *Nursing Medical Emergency Patients*. London, Wiley-Blackwell.

Department of Health (2000) *Comprehensive Critical Care – A Review of Adult Critical Care Services*. London, Department of Health.

Dracup K (1995) *Meltzer's Intensive Coronary Care: A Manual for Nurses* (5e). London, Prentice Hall International (UK).

Gao H, McDonnell A, Harrison DA *et al.* (2007) Systematic review and evaluation of physiological track and trigger warning systems for identifying at-risk patients on the ward. *Intensive Care Medicine* **33**: 667–79.

Kumar P and Clark M (2000) *Clinical Medicine* (5e). London, Saunders.

Haig KM, Sutton S and Whittington J (2006) SBAR: A shared mental model for improving communication between clinicians. *Joint Commission Journal on Quality and Patient Safety* **32**(3):167–75.

Humphreys M (2009) Cardiac emergencies. In: Jevon P, Humphreys M and Ewens B (eds) (2009) *Nursing Medical Emergency Patients*. London, Wiley-Blackwell.

Humphreys M (2006) Pericardial conditions: signs, symptoms and electrocardiogram changes. *Emergency Nurse* **14**(1): 30–6.

Lilly LS (1998) *Pathophysiology of Heart Disease: A Collaborative Project of Medical students and faculty* (2e). London, Lea & Febiger.

McConachie I and Roberts H (2000) *Handbook of Cardiac Emergencies.* London, Greenwich Medical Media.

McCance KL and Huether SE (1998) *Pathophysiology: The Biologic Basis for Disease in Adults and Children* (3e). St Louis, Mosby Yearbook.

McGaughey J (2009) *Outreach and Early Warning Systems (EWS) for the Prevention of Intensive Care Admission and Death of Critically Ill Adult Patients on General Hospital Wards.* The Cochrane Collaboration, John Wiley & Sons. Available at http://mrw.interscience.wiley.com/cochrane/clsysrev/articles/CD005529/frame.html

Millane T, Jackson G, Gibbs CR and Lip GYH (2000) ABC of heart failure. Acute and chronic management strageties. *British Medical Journal* **320**(7228): 559-62.

Myerson S, Choudhury R and Mitchell A (2010) *Emergencies in Cardiology* (2e). Oxford, Oxford University Press.

NICE (2007) *Acutely Ill Patients in Hospital: Recognition of and Response to Acute Illness in Adults in Hospital.* Clinical Guideline 50. London. NICE:

National Confidential Enquiry into Patient Outcome and Death (NCEPOD) (2005) *An Acute Problem?* London, NCEPOD.

National Patient Safety Agency (NPSA) (2007) *Recognising and Responding Appropriately to Early Signs of Deterioration in Hospitalised Patients.* London, NPSA.

Nolan J, Grewood J and Mackintosh A (1998) *Cardiac Emergencies: A Pocket Guide.* Oxford, Butterworth Heinemann.

Porth CM (1994) *Pathophysiology: Concepts of Altered Health States* (4e). Philadelphia, Lippincott.

Resuscitation Council UK (2010) *Advanced Life Support Provider Manual* (6e). London, Resuscitation Council UK.

Rose B and Post T (2005) *Clinical Physiology of Acid-Base and Electrolyte Disorders* (5e). London, McGraw-Hill Medical.

Smith G (2003) *ALERT – Acute Life Threatening Events Recognition and Treatment* (2e). Portsmouth, University of Portsmouth.

Souhami R and Moxham J (2002) *Textbook of Medicine* (4e). London, Churchill Livingstone.

Sprigings DC and Chambers JB (2001) *Acute Medicine: A Practical Guide to the Management of Medical Emergencies.* Oxford, Blackwell Science.

Thompson PL (2005) *Coronary Care Manual* (2e). London, Churchill Livingstone.

Tortora G and Derrickson B (2008) *Principles of Anatomy and Physiology* (12e). Philadelphia, John Wiley and Sons.

Wyatt J, Illingworth R, Clancy M and Robertson C (1998) *Oxford Handbook of Accident and Emergency Medicine.* Oxford, Oxford University Press.

Chapter 12
Long-Term Cardiac Conditions

Ian Jones and Anne Dormer

Introduction

It is estimated that by 2025 there will be 18 million people in the UK affected by a long-term illness (DH, 2007). Consequently the government has made supporting people with a long-term condition a priority for health and social care; with particular emphasis on prevention, early detection and management, cardiac conditions feature largely within this agenda. The Public Service Agreement (PSA) targets (DH, 2004) sought to improve the health outcomes for people with long-term conditions by offering a personalised care plan for vulnerable people most at risk and improving access to services.

These aims have been incorporated into a new strategic model to support people through all stages of their condition (National Service Framework [NSF] for long-term conditions [LTC]; DH, 2005a), which focuses on improving self-care, disease control and management of their condition. Central to this model is the individual being an active participant in all decisions relating to their care (DH, 2001). Many specialty clinics are nurse-led and nurses are acquiring advanced knowledge and skills to be able to work effectively in this new milieu. Specialist roles are rapidly developing to meet the service requirements of cardiac patients with long-term conditions. Nurses specialising in heart failure, cardiomyopathy, chronic pain and arrhythmias are currently forging links between all sectors of health and social care. Patients with cardiac problems are also living longer, the nurse's role in end-of-life care is gaining momentum, and cardiac nurses are already developing roles and expertise in palliative care. The aim of this chapter is to enhance evidence-based knowledge and analytical skills in assessing, planning, implementing and evaluating care that the individual person and their family/carer receive in relation to the management of their long-term cardiac condition.

Nursing the Cardiac Patient, First Edition. Edited by Melanie Humphreys.
© 2011 Blackwell Publishing Ltd. Published 2011 by Blackwell Publishing Ltd.

Learning outcomes

At the end of this chapter the reader will be able to:

- describe the prevalence of long-term cardiac illness
- identify the causes of long-term cardiac diseases
- discuss the evidence-based management of patients living with a long-term cardiac condition.

Heart failure

Heart failure is a common clinical syndrome that results from any structural or functional cardiac disorder that impairs the pumping ability of the heart, and it represents the end point of many cardiovascular diseases (Cowie *et al.*, 2000). The annual incidence of this condition is estimated to be around 0.3% (McDonagh and Dargie 1998) and it is prevalent in between 0.9% (Cowie *et al.*, 1999) and 1.8% (Davies *et al.*, 2001) of the general UK population. The prevalence of heart failure also increases with older age. Indeed, it is projected that both the number of people diagnosed with heart failure and hospital admissions for heart failure will increase significantly over the next 20–30 years (Stewart *et al.*, 2003; Gnani and Ellis, 2001). This is due to the ageing population in the UK and also is a result of success in managing coronary heart disease (CHD). However, many people surviving myocardial infarction (MI) will live with damaged hearts that will, over time, progress to heart failure.

Heart failure is a progressive and largely unpredictable condition. As a consequence, heart failure patients experience significant changes that affect their quality of life (Moser and Dracup, 2001). Many patients with heart failure will deteriorate over a two- to five-year period. Their illness will normally be characterised by organ system failure and increasing debility, often accompanied by more frequent "acute" episodes of illness sometimes requiring hospital admission (Thompson, 2007). It is also known from epidemiological studies that once heart failure is diagnosed mortality rates are high. The Hillingdon Heart Failure study (Cowie *et al.*, 2000) found that 43% of patients with heart failure had died within 18 months of diagnosis.

Causes of heart failure

The underlying cause/aetiology of heart failure should be identified to ensure correct patient management and optimum treatment.

The commonest cause of heart failure in Europe is myocardial dysfunction secondary to coronary artery disease, resulting in left ventricular (LV) systolic dysfunction (European Society of Cardiology, 2008). Around two-thirds of cases of heart failure are attributable to coronary artery disease.

The remainder have non-ischaemic systolic dysfunction, which may be due to one of the following causes (Davies *et al.*, 2006):

- hypertension
- valvular or congenital heart disease
- alcohol or the toxic effect of drugs
- high output failure, e.g. thyroid disease or anaemia
- arrhythmias – atrial fibrillation (AF), tachycardia, bradycardia
- pericardial disease
- primary right heart failure as a result of pulmonary embolism or cor pulmonale.

Diagnosing heart failure

Diagnosing heart failure is challenging for the clinician as many other conditions share similar signs and symptoms.

For a diagnosis of heart failure criteria 1 and 2 should be fulfilled in all cases:

1 symptoms of heart failure
2 objective evidence of cardiac dysfunction, and in cases where there is doubt
3 response to treatment directed towards heart failure.
   (European Society of Heart Failure, 2001)

Breathlessness, fatigue and reduced exercise tolerance are frequently reported in heart failure. The New York Heart Association classification of symptoms is universally used to quantify a patient's functional capacity and is determined by an assessment of symptoms as reported by the patient (Box 12.1).

Symptoms in heart failure
- Dyspnoea
- Orthopnoea
- Paroxysmal nocturnal dyspnoea
- Reduced exercise tolerance, lethargy and fatigue
- Nocturnal cough
- Wheeze
- Ankle swelling, leg oedema, abdominal distension
- Anorexia
- Mental effects – depression

Signs in heart failure
- Pulse – tachycardia, may be irregular
- Blood pressure – may be low
- Jugular venous pressure (JVP) – may be elevated

Box 12.1 The New York Heart Association (CCNYHA, 1994) classification of heart failure

NYHA I

Patients have no limitation on activities and experience no symptoms from ordinary activities; however, there is evidence of left ventricular impairment on echocardiography.

NYHA II

Patients experience mild limitation of activity; they are comfortable at rest or with mild exertion. Evidence of mild to moderate left ventricular impairment on echocardiography.

NYHA III

Patients experience marked limitation of activity; they are comfortable only at rest. Evidence of moderate to severe left ventricular impairment on echocardiography.

NYHA IV

Patients confined to bed or chair; even minimal activity causes discomfort and symptoms occur at rest. Evidence of severe left ventricular impairment on echocardiography.

(Criteria Committee of the New York Heart Association, 1994; in Cowie, 2005)

- Displaced apex beat
- Extra heart sound, e.g. third heart sound, gallop rhythm
- Right ventricular heave
- Lungs – crepitations or wheeze
- Oedema – peripheral, sacral
- Cachexia and muscle wasting

It is important that the practitioner investigates the patient to exclude other conditions that may present with similar symptoms to heart failure, which include (NICE, 2010):

- obesity
- chest disease
- venous insufficiency in lower limbs
- drug-induced ankle swelling, e.g. dihydropyridine calcium channel blockers

- drug-induced fluid congestion, e.g. non-steroidal anti-inflammatory drugs (NSAIDs)
- hypoalbuminaemia
- intrinsic renal or hepatic disease
- pulmonary embolic disease
- depression/anxiety disorders
- severe anaemia or thyroid disease
- bilateral renal artery stenosis.

Investigations

For patients with suspected heart failure the following investigations should be undertaken to exclude differential diagnoses and to determine the patients need for echocardiogram.

Electrocardiography

The 12-lead ECG is abnormal in most patients with heart failure, although it may be normal in 10% of cases (Davies *et al.*, 2000).

Common abnormalities include:

- Q waves
- ST segment abnormalities
- atrial fibrillation
- left bundle branch block
- left ventricular hypertrophy.

B-type natriuretic peptide (BNP)

Plasma BNP and NT-proBNP are hormones produced by the heart as a result of ventricular stress. Levels are elevated in patients with heart failure, therefore patients with a normal BNP or NT-proBNP level may be excluded from the diagnosis of heart failure. An abnormal NT-proBNP concentration is an accurate diagnostic test both for the exclusion of heart failure in the population and in ruling out LV dysfunction in breathless individuals (McDonagh *et al.*, 2004).

Chest X-ray

A chest X-ray is a useful test to observe for evidence of:

- cardiomegaly (an enlarged heart)
- pulmonary oedema (fluid on the lungs)
- lung disease that may cause breathlessness.

Spirometry

Assessment and evaluation of pulmonary function is useful to exclude lung disease as a cause of breathlessness.

Blood tests

The following blood tests are recommended as part of a routine diagnostic evaluation of patients with suspected heart failure (European Society of Cardiology, 2001):

- full blood count – exclude anaemia as a cause of heart failure
- urea and electrolytes
- fasting glucose and lipid profile
- liver function tests
- thyroid function test – exclude thyroid disease as a cause of heart failure
- C-reactive protein
- uric acid.

In the case of an acute presentation of breathlessness/chest pain, myocardial infarction should be excluded (*see* Chapter 3).

Echocardiography

Transthoracic Doppler echocardiography is the gold standard test for the diagnosis of heart failure. It is a safe and reliable test if performed by suitably trained operators and is widely available.

Echocardiography enables visualisation of the cardiac walls, chambers and valves, and identifies patients with left ventricular systolic dysfunction (LVSD), giving an estimate of the left ventricular ejection fraction.

SIGN guidance (2007) recommends that the echocardiograph investigation should include:

- a description of overall left ventricular systolic function together with any wall motion abnormalities
- assessment of diastolic function
- measurement of left ventricular wall thickness
- Doppler assessment of any significant valve disease
- estimation of pulmonary artery systolic pressure, where possible (*see* Figure 12.1).

Pharmacology therapy

Pharmacological therapy is the cornerstone of management in chronic heart failure. Compensatory mechanisms are activated in heart failure to preserve cardiac function, in particular the renin–aldosterone–angiotensin system (RAAS) and the sympathetic nervous system (SNS). The use of angiotensin-converting enzyme inhibitors, beta-blockers and aldosterone antagonists have demonstrated their effectiveness in improving symptoms and patient survival by regulating the harmful effects of the RAAS and SNS systems.

- *ACE inhibitors* are accepted as standard treatment and should be considered in patients with all functional classes of heart failure due to LVSD.

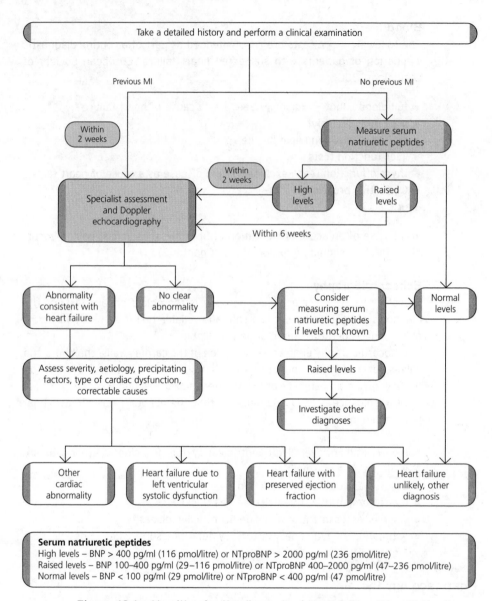

Take a detailed history and perform a clinical examination

Previous MI

No previous MI

Within 2 weeks

Measure serum natriuretic peptides

Within 2 weeks

High levels

Raised levels

Specialist assessment and Doppler echocardiography

Within 6 weeks

Abnormality consistent with heart failure

No clear abnormality

Consider measuring serum natriuretic peptides if levels not known

Normal levels

Assess severity, aetiology, precipitating factors, type of cardiac dysfunction, correctable causes

Raised levels

Investigate other diagnoses

Other cardiac abnormality

Heart failure due to left ventricular systolic dysfunction

Heart failure with preserved ejection fraction

Heart failure unlikely, other diagnosis

Serum natriuretic peptides
High levels – BNP > 400 pg/ml (116 pmol/litre) or NTproBNP > 2000 pg/ml (236 pmol/litre)
Raised levels – BNP 100–400 pg/ml (29–116 pmol/litre) or NTproBNP 400–2000 pg/ml (47–236 pmol/litre)
Normal levels – BNP < 100 pg/ml (29 pmol/litre) or NTproBNP < 400 pg/ml (47 pmol/litre)

Figure 12.1 Algorithm for the diagnosis of heart failure. From National Institute Clinical Excellence (2010). Reproduced with permission.

ACE inhibitors have demonstrated in large clinical trials improvement in symptoms, exercise tolerance, mortality rates and readmissions to hospital. For those patients intolerant of an ACE inhibitor, an angiotensin receptor blocker should be considered (NICE, 2010).

- *Diuretic therapy* is necessary to relieve breathlessness and oedema secondary to fluid congestion. Loop diuretics are the usual agent of choice (e.g. furosemide or bumetanide). In patients with advanced heart failure who demonstrate resistant fluid retention, adding in a thiazide diuretic may be considered. This is known as combination therapy. Care should be taken to use the lowest dose possible to relieve symptoms without side effects, e.g. dehydration and/or renal dysfunction.

- *Beta-blockers* should be prescribed to all patients with heart failure due to LVSD as soon as their condition is stable. Bisoprolol, carvedilol and nebivolol are the beta-blockers of choice (SIGN, 2007). Large-scale clinical trials have demonstrated improvements in quality of life, symptoms, and mortality and readmission rates.
- The *angiotensin receptor blocker* candesartan should be considered as add-on therapy for patients already tolerating an ACE inhibitor and other standard therapies but who remain moderately to severely symptomatic (SIGN, 2007).
- The *aldosterone antagonist* spironolactone is indicated for patients with moderate to severe heart failure (NYHA III-IV). Pitt *et al.* (1999) demonstrated spironolactone in moderate to severe heart failure reduced all cause and cardiac mortality, with reduction in readmissions to hospital, when added to standard therapy.
- *Digoxin* does not offer improved survival in heart failure. Digoxin may be initially used for rate control in AF but use of a beta-blocker for rate control is advised (SIGN, 2007).

Lifestyle advice/self-management

Education and counselling is essential to empower the patient to self-manage their condition and comply with prescribed therapies.

Exercise
Heart failure patients should be encouraged to adopt regular, low-intensity physical activity (NICE, 2010). Regular activity benefits patient outcomes by improving symptoms, improving patient sense of wellbeing, and increasing energy levels and functional capacity.

Salt and fluid restriction
A high-salt diet may lead to fluid retention. Patients should be advised to avoid highly salted foods and not to add salt to their food at the table. The Food Standards Agency recommends that the total salt intake for adults should not exceed 6 g per day. Heart failure patients should be advised not to use low-salt substitutes because of their higher potassium content.

Fluid restrictions may be recommended for individual patients with severe symptoms and signs of fluid congestion. Symptomatic patients may be advised to limit their fluid intake to 1.5–2 l daily. High fluid intake negates the positive effect of diuretic therapy and may lead to hyponatraemia (Davies, 2009).

Nutrition

Heart failure patients have increased nutritional requirements due to an increase in metabolic rate (Davies, 2009: p.26). However, patients with advanced heart failure are at risk of malnutrition if there is reduction in appetite, malabsorption problems, anorexia or nausea. This may lead to cardiac cachexia manifested by muscle wasting. Small regular portions of high-energy foods should be offered in conjunction with nutritional assessment by a dietician.

Home daily weight monitoring

Patients with chronic heart failure should be encouraged to weigh themselves regularly, particularly those with a previous history of fluid congestion. Patients should keep a record of their weight taken at the same time of day, before dressing. A weight gain of 2 kg over two days or 4 kg over one week should be reported to their GP or heart failure practitioner, particularly if associated with worsening symptoms.

Smoking

Patients with chronic heart failure should be strongly advised not to smoke. Smoking cessation is a very difficult lifestyle change to make, therefore advice and support should be offered to the patient.

Alcohol consumption

All patients with heart failure should be encouraged to refrain from excessive alcohol consumption, as alcohol is a myocardial depressant and has direct toxic effects on the myocardium.

Immunisation

The flu virus and chest infection may exacerbate heart failure. Patients should be offered an annual influenza immunisation and a once-only pneumococcal immunisation (NICE, 2010).

Contraceptive advice

In women of childbearing age contraceptive advice should be offered, as there is a high incidence of increased heart failure symptoms in pregnancy and increased maternal mortality in women with significant left ventricular dysfunction.

Anxiety and depression

Anxiety and/or depression following a diagnosis of heart failure is common and use of a screening tool such as the Hospital Anxiety and Depression Scale (Zigmond and Snaith, 1983) may help to identify patients who are affected. Referral to clinical psychology may be indicated if such a service is available in the locality. Otherwise, the ability to talk to a knowledgeable key worker and/or prescription of a suitable antidepressant may be helpful.

Depression is a recognised poor prognostic indicator in cardiac disease (Faris *et al.*, 2002; Vaccarino *et al.*, 2001).

Device therapy and surgical interventions

Implantable cardioverter defibrillators and cardiac re-synchronisation therapy

Implantable cardioverter defibrillators (ICD) are used to treat patients at risk of ventricular arrhythmias and are therefore an important part of the management of heart failure patients; their use is two-fold: in secondary and primary prevention (Boxes 12.2 and 12.3).

Cardiac resynchronisation therapy (CRT) is a treatment using a pacemaker in specific heart failure patients. It improves the function of the heart by ensuring the ventricles contract at the same time (synchrony). A left bundle branch block pattern on ECG may indicate cardiac dyssynchrony. Cardiac dyssynchrony is associated with reduced pump efficiency and may lead increasing heart failure symptoms such as breathlessness (Box 12.4).

Cardiac resynchronisation therapy is used to restore timing or synchrony of ventricular contraction and improve pump efficiency. The CRT pacemaker has three pacing leads. One lead is placed in the right atria and one in the right ventricle, like a standard pacemaker. In CRT pacemakers a third pacing lead is inserted into one of the coronary veins via the coronary sinus, which enables pacing of the left ventricle, improving timing of the left and right ventricular contraction and of the walls of the left ventricle. CRT can also improve atrio-ventricular timing.

Recommendations for other surgical interventions include left ventricular assist device and cardiac transplantation. Patients in severe heart failure

---

Box 12.2   Secondary prevention: implantable cardioverter defibrillators

Secondary prevention – patients presenting, in the absence of a reversible cause, with one of the following.

- Having survived a cardiac arrest due to either ventricular tachycardia (VT) or ventricular fibrillation (VF).
- Spontaneous sustained VT causing syncope or significant haemodynamic compromise.
- Sustained VT without syncope or cardiac arrest, and who have an associated reduction in ejection fraction (LVEF <35%) and are no worse than NYHA class III.

From National Institute for Health and Clinical Excellence (2006). Reproduced with permission.

> ### Box 12.3 Primary prevention: implantable cardioverter defibrillators
>
> Primary prevention – patients with a history of MI (more than 4 weeks) and either:
>
> - LVSD with an ejection fraction <35% (no worse than NYHA class III) and
> - non-sustained VT on 24 h ECG (NSVT is three or more consecutive ventricular beats at a rate of greater than 120 beats/min with a duration of less than 30 s) and
> - inducible VT on electrophysiological (EP) testing
>
> OR
>
> - LVSD with an ejection fraction <30% (no worse than NYHA class III)
> - QRS duration of equal to or more than 120 ms.
>
> From National Institute for Health and Clinical Excellence (2006). Reproduced with permission.

> ### Box 12.4 Definition of dyssynchrony
>
> What is dyssynchrony?
>
> - The loss of synchronised contraction between left and right ventricles (interventricular).
> - The loss of synchronised contraction of the left ventricular walls (intraventricular).
> - It is caused by interruption of the ventricular conduction system and is seen on electrocardiogram as a broad complex QRS >120 ms.

despite optimal therapy should be referred to an advanced heart failure centre where they may be assessed for left ventricular assist device as a bridge to transplantation or their suitability for cardiac transplantation.

Refractory angina

Prevalence

Angina pectoris is a common condition that affects approximately 2% of the general population (Stewart et al., 2002) and has been noted as high as 7%

in a cohort over the age of 45 years (Cosin *et al.*, 1999). The majority of these patients will be managed effectively using a combination of pharmacological and interventional treatments. However, a growing number of patients are either, unable to receive, or are resistant to, conventional medical therapy. It has been estimated that this figure may be as high as 15% of the angina population (Mannheimer *et al.*, 2002) and is likely to increase further as the mortality rates from acute coronary syndromes continue to fall.

Definition

This condition has been assigned many different titles, including intractable angina, end-stage heart disease and refractory angina. However, Mannheimer *et al.* (2002), in their report for the European Society of Cardiology, argue that the terms intractable angina and end-stage heart disease are misleading as they suggest that the condition is not accessible to further treatment. The Society has therefore adopted the standard term of refractory angina, which they define as "a chronic condition characterised by the presence of angina caused by coronary insufficiency in the presence of coronary artery disease which cannot be controlled by a combination of medical therapy, angioplasty and coronary artery bypass surgery". This definition recognises that alternative treatments may produce beneficial effects for the patient

Without such treatment the patients often find their symptoms disabling. Their chronic chest pain can often give rise to poor sleep patterns, and anxiety and depression. It can also leave them physically inactive and socially isolated (Lewin *et al.*, 2002; Lewin, 1999). It is therefore imperative that these patients receive a thorough assessment by a trained cardiologist and cardiac surgeon prior to treatment being considered.

Assessment

This assessment should include an appraisal of the patient's medical history, physical examination and a review of current medications. The practitioner should first rule out any differential diagnosis and non-cardiac causes such as costochondritis and thyrotoxicosis (*see* Chapter 3). The practitioner would need to ensure that the patient was receiving the optimal dosages of prescribed therapy (*see* Chapter 5), and this should be titrated accordingly.

The cardiologist may undertake additional investigations (e.g. angiography) to confirm the presence of cardiac disease and identify areas of disease that may be treatable. In the event of these investigations confirming a diagnosis of refractory angina, there are a number of therapies available, unfortunately many of these interventions remain in the early stages of their development and have yet to develop an established evidence base.

Treatment

The approaches currently advocated are not without debate as to effectiveness and need to be investigated further before they can be accepted as viable therapy choices for the management of this group, but they include:

- enhanced external counter pulsation
- nerve stimulation
- myocardial revascularisation
- angiogenesis.

There are a number of additional therapies that are currently being considered to reduce the symptom burden of patients with refractory angina, but at present many of these interventions lack the evidence to support their inclusion in routine care.

Nursing management

While many of these therapies are invasive and indeed traumatic, it should be remembered that there are a number of interventions that are less intrusive and may be equally or even more effective. Patients who suffer from refractory angina often experience a markedly reduced quality of life and may suffer from anxiety and depression. Nurses can play a key role in addressing many of these issues and referring the patient for cardiac rehabilitation sessions (see Chapters 13 and 14). Patients with refractory angina often become physically inactive, which in turn may lead to weight gain, but this inactivity if reversed can increase the angina threshold by increasing the efficacy of the musculoskeletal system. As a result, the patient will be able to undertake more of their daily activities without experiencing chest pain.

Due to the costs involved, refractory angina is a growing concern for all healthcare markets, and while professional groups provide management guidance there is a lack of evidence available to support any single strategy. It is therefore clear that there is an urgent need to study the efficacy of both invasive treatments and nurse-led interventions in this group. Without such evidence the management of these patients will remain suboptimal.

Atrial fibrillation

Definition

Atrial fibrillation is a supraventricular tachyarrhythmia resulting in uncoordinated atrial activation and deterioration of atrial function (Fuster *et al.*, 2006). It is characterised on the ECG as an absence of P waves and irregular ventricular complexes that occur as a result of multiple re-entry circuits within the atrial tissue (Figure 12.2). It can be characterised as paroxysmal, persistent or permanent in nature, and is the most common sustainable arrhythmia encountered in cardiac care (National Collaborating Centre for

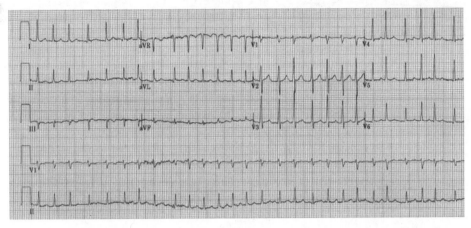

Figure 12.2 12 Lead ECG showing atrial fibrillation. Fibrillatory waves are best seen in leads II and V₁.

Chronic Conditions, 2006). The term paroxysmal refers to the episodic nature of the condition, whereas permanent refers to the fact that the AF is sustained despite previous cardioversion, or where cardioversion has not been attempted. Persistent AF is diagnosed when the rhythm has persisted beyond 7 days but has not been treated (Humphreys, 2001).

Prevalence

Atrial fibrillation occurs in 1% of the population, rising to 4% in people aged 45 years (DH, 2005b), and is as high as 10% in those over the age of 75 years (Lip and Lim, 2007). Atrial fibrillation is not a benign condition. The symptoms alone affect the quality of life of two-thirds of those with the condition (Wyse *et al.*, 2002), but it is perhaps the risk of stroke that makes AF such an important condition. This risk varies, but if AF is left untreated the risk of stroke increases fivefold (Markides and Schilling, 2003), and the risk of all-cause mortality is double that of patients in sinus rhythm (Krahn *et al.*, 1995; Flegel *et al.*, 1987; Kannel *et al.*, 1983).

Assessment

Chapter 8 of the National Service Framework for coronary heart disease (DH, 2005b) stated that people presenting with arrhythmias, in both emergency and elective settings, should receive timely assessment by an appropriate clinician to ensure accurate diagnosis and effective treatment and rehabilitation.

This statement recognises the need for patients with AF to be identified early and treated appropriately. However, the decision-making process is dependent on a number of factors. The cause of AF is a fundamental question that needs to be posed. Many causes of AF, such as alcohol intake and thyrotoxicosis, are reversible. In such cases the successful treatment of the underlying cause can lead to elimination of the arrhythmia. However, AF also occurs in the presence of cardiovascular disease such as mitral valve disease, coronary heart disease and cardiomyopathy. Consequently, a review of a patient with suspected AF needs to include a 12-lead ECG, full medical history to establish the sustainability, tolerability and prior management of the arrhythmia, and additional investigations to identify possible causes of the AF (Box 12.5).

Once a diagnosis of AF is confirmed the practitioner needs to consider both the effects of treatment on underlying medical conditions such as heart failure and the risk of stroke. The latter is achieved using a risk stratification formula such as the CHADS2 score (Gage et al., 2001).

Treatment

Once identified, all patients should receive a hard copy of their ECG documenting their arrhythmia, and a copy should be placed in their records (DH, 2005b).

The goal for the management of AF should be either to attempt to return the patient to a normal sinus rhythm or reduce the heart rate. The former can be achieved either chemically using drugs such as amiodarone, electrically through DC cardioversion or electrophysiologically through surgical or catheter ablation. The latter strategy is adopted to reduce the risks associated with tachycardias, such as heart failure. In this latter approach the patient will continue to experience AF but at a lower ventricular rate. However, it should be noted that all patients with symptomatic AF despite optimal medical therapy should be referred to a heart rhythm specialist (DH 2005b).

The National Institute for Health and Clinical Excellence (2006) provides clinical guidelines for the management of patients with AF. They recommend that patients with paroxysmal AF should be considered primarily for cardioversion. The way in which the restoration of normal rhythm is to be achieved is one for discussion between the practitioner and the patient, taking into account the merits of both chemical and DC cardioversion. However, they suggest that prolonged AF (>48h) should be treated with electrical cardioversion.

The most complex group are those patients suffering from persistent AF. The NICE guidelines (2006) acknowledge the numerous clinical trials that have explored this phenomenon have not demonstrated a superior strategy. However, the guidelines advise when rate or rhythm control is preferred (Box 12.6). Due to the risk of stroke antithrombotic treatment should be considered regardless of approach.

Nursing management

Nurses have a key role to play in identifying and caring for patients with AF. This role takes many forms and can occur in different settings. The primary

Box 12.5   Investigations for the patient with atrial fibrillation

History and physical examination to include:

- Symptom assessment
- Blood pressure
- Clinical type of AF (persistent, paroxysmal, permanent)
- Onset of first attack and duration
- Precipitating factors and modes of termination
- Response to any drugs administered
- Presence of underlying condition or reversible cause

ECG

- Rhythm
- LV hypertrophy
- Pre-excitation
- Bundle branch block
- Previous MI
- P wave duration and fibrillatory waves
- Other arrhythmias
- Monitor waveform intervals in conjunction with therapy

Transthoracic echocardiogram

- Valve disease
- LA and RA size
- LV size and function
- RV pressure
- LV hypertrophy
- Thrombus
- Pericardial disease

Blood tests

- Full blood count
- Urea and electrolytes
- Thyroid function
- Clotting screen
- Glucose

Further tests may be required.

Box 12.6 Distinguishing between rate versus rhythm control

Rate control preferred if:

- Over 65
- Presence of coronary disease
- Contraindications to anti arrhythmic therapy
- Unsuitable for cardioversion
- Without heart failure

Rhythm control preferred if:

- Symptomatic
- Younger patients
- First-time presentation
- Secondary to a treatable condition
- Congestive heart failure

care role may include the identification of AF in those at-risk groups and the regular review of patients living with AF. This review should include an assessment of the patient's current risk of stroke and other complications of the condition. The nurse should also consider the patient's understanding of their illness and their concordance with treatment.

Acute care nurses may identify the presence of AF during a paroxysmal episode or as part of a routine patient assessment. However, the latter is less likely if nurses rely on machinery as opposed to the traditional but still the most informative means of checking heart rate that is the pulse check. While the management of these situations will differ according to the classification of the condition, the identification of AF in any patient should be considered an important finding that warrants further investigation and treatment.

More specialist nurses have taken a lead in co-ordinating specific AF clinics. There is a wealth of evidence to demonstrate that these clinics provide an effective means of identifying, risk stratifying and treating patients with AF. They also demonstrate that nurses provide effective clinical care and co-ordination of the services regardless of their setting (Smallwood, 2005; Currie et al., 2004; Quinn, 1999).

Summary

There is no doubt that the number of people living with long-term cardiac conditions will increase dramatically over the next decade. While the reductions in mortality from acute heart disease and other common diseases has enabled people to live longer, many of these people will live the remainder of their lives with complex health problems.

It is therefore essential that cardiac nurses possess a deep understanding of the long-term management of their patients and the strategies required to care for them. Unlike acute care, where patients are continually observed, patients with long-term conditions will not have constant access to a health-care professional. Yet they remain at risk of deterioration and suffering further complications of their condition. It is therefore imperative that people living with long-term conditions are provided with the information and support they require to take control of their healthcare and make informed decisions about that care. As a consequence they are more likely to be con-cordant with their drug regimen and recognise changes in their condition, which would allow early intervention.

Unlike acute care, where the predominant aim is to maintain life, the aim of long-term care should be to maintain the quality of that life for as long as possible. This can only be achieved if the nurse adopts the role of supportive partner rather than paternalistic care provider.

References

Cosın J, Asın E, Marrugat J et al. (1999) Prevalence of angina pectoris in Spain. PANES Study group. *European Journal of Epidemiology* **4**: 323-30.

Cowie M (2005) Clinical background: heart failure and implementation of the NICE/NCC-CC guideline. In: *Managing Chronic Heart Failure: Learning from Best Practice*. London, Clinical Effectiveness and Evaluation Unit, Royal College of Physicians, p.1.

Cowie M, Wood D, Coates A et al. (2000) Survival of patients with a new diagnosis of heart failure: a population based study. *Heart* **83**: 505-10.

Cowie MR, Wood DA, Coats AJS et al. (1999) Incidence and aetiology of heart failure: a population based study. *European Heart Journal* **20**(6): 421-8.

Currie MP, Karwatowski SP, Perera J and Langford EJ (2004) Introduction of a nurse led DC cardioversion service in day surgery unit: prospective audit. *British Medical Journal* **329**: 892-4.

Davies A (2009) Permanent pacemakers: an overview. *British Journal of Cardiac Nursing* **4**(6): 262-9.

Davies MK, Hobbs FDR, Davies RC et al. (2001) Prevalence of left ventricular systolic dysfunction and heart failure in the echocardiographic Heart of England Study: a population based study. *Lancet* **358**: 439-44.

Davies RC, Davies MK, Lip GYH (2006) *ABC of Heart Failure* (2e). Oxford, Blackwell Publishing/BMJ Books.

Davies RC, Gibbs CR and Lip GYH (2000) Investigation. In: Gibbs CR, Davies MK and Lip GYH *ABC of Heart Failure*. London, BMJ Books.

Department of Health (2007) *Raising the Profile of Long Term Conditions Care. A Compendium of Information*. London, Department of Health.

Department of Health (2005a) *The National Service Framework (NSF) for Long-term Conditions*. London, Department of Health.

Department of Health (2005b) *National Service Framework for Coronary Heart Disease. Chapter 8: Arrhythmias and Sudden Cardiac Death*. London, Department of Health.

Department of Health (2004) *National Standards and Local Action Health and Social Care Standards and Planning Framework 2005/06-2007/08*. London, Department of Health.

Department of Health (2001) *The Expert Patient: A New Approach to Chronic Disease*. London, Department of Health.

European Society of Cardiology (ESC) (2008) Task force report guidelines for the diagnosis and treatment of chronic heart failure. *European Heart Journal* **22**: 1527-60.

Faris R, Purcell H, Henien M and Coats A (2002) Clinical depression is common and significantly associated with reduced survival in non ischaemic heart failure. *European Journal of Heart Failure* **4**(4): 541-51.

Flegel KM, Shipley MJ and Rose G (1987). Risk of stroke in non-rheumatic atrial fibrillation. *Lancet* **1**(878): 526-9.

Fuster V, Ryden LE, Cannom DS *et al.* for the American College of Cardiology/American Heart Association Task Force on Practice Guidelines and the European Society of Cardiology Committee for Practice Guidelines (2006) ACC/AHA/ESC 2006 Guidelines for the management of patients with atrial fibrillation. *Circulation* **114**(7): e257-354.

Gage BF, Waterman AD, Shannon W, Boechler M, Rich MW and Radford MJ (2001) Validation of clinical classifi cation schemes for predicting stroke: results from the National Registry of Atrial Fibrillation. *Journal of the American Medical Association* **285**(22): 2864-70.

Gnani S and Ellis C (2001) Trends in hospital admissions and cased fatality due to heart failure in England, 1990/91 to 1999/2000. *Health Statistics Quarterly* **13**: 16-21.

Humphreys M (2001) Atrial fibrillation: the most common form of arrhythmia. *Connect: Critical Care Nursing in Europe* **1**(3): 93-6.

Kannel WB, Abbott RD, Savage DD *et al.* (1983) Coronary heart disease and atrial fibrillation: the Framingham Study. *American Heart Journal* **106**: 389-96.

Krahn AD, Manfreda J, Tate RB *et al.* (1995). The natural history of atrial fibrillation: incidence, risk factors, and prognosis in the Manitoba Follow-Up Study. *American Journal of Medicine* **98**: 476-84.

Lewin RJ (1999) Improving quality of life in patients with angina. *Heart* **82**: 654-5.

Lewin RJ, Furze G, Robinson J *et al.* (2002) A randomised controlled trial of a self-management plan for patients with newly diagnosed angina. *British Journal of General Practice* **52**: 194-201.

Lip GYH and Lim HS (2007) Atrial fibrillation and stroke prevention. *Lancet Neurology* **6**: 981-93.

Mannheimer C, Camici P, Chester MR *et al.* (2002) The problem of chronic refractory angina: report from the ESC Joint Study Group on the Treatment of Refractory Angina. *European Heart Journal* **23**: 355-70.

Markides V and Schilling R (2003) Atrial fibrillation: classification, pathophysiology, mechanisms and drug treatment. *Heart* **89**: 939-43.

McDonagh TA and Dargie ,H J (1998) Epidemiology and pathophysiology of heart failure. *Medicine* **26**: 111-15.

McDonagh TA, Homer S, Raymond I, Luchner A, Hildebrant P and Dargie HJ (2004) NT-proBNP and the diagnosis of heart failure: a pooled analysis of three European epidemiological studies. *European Journal of Heart Failure* **6**: 269-73.

Moser DK and Dracup K (2001) Impact of nonpharmacologic therapy on quality of life in heart failure. In: Moser DK and Riegel B *Improving Outcomes in Heart Failure: An Interdisciplinary Approach*. Maryland, Aspen Publishers.

National Collaborating Centre for Chronic Conditions (2006) *Atrial Fibrillation: National Clinical Guidelines for Management in Primary and Secondary Care* (NICE Clinical Guideline 36). London, Royal College of Physicians.

National Institute Clinical Excellence (2010) *CG 108 Chronic Heart Failure: Management of Chronic Heart Failure in Adults in Primary and Secondary Care*. London, NICE. Available from www.nice.org.uk/CG108

National Institute for Health and Clinical Excellence (2006) *TA 95 Implantable cardioverter defibrillators for arrhythmias*. London, NICE. Available from www.nice.org.uk/TA95

Pitt B, Zannad F, Remme WJ *et al.* (1999) The effect of spironolactone on morbidity and mortality in patients with severe heart failure. Randomised Aldactone Evaluation Study Investigators. *New England Journal of Medicine* **341**: 709-77.

Quinn T (1998) Early experience of nurse-led elective DC cardioversion. *Nursing in Critical Care* **3**(2): 59-62.

Scottish Intercollegiate Guideline Network (SIGN) (2007) Management of Chronic Heart Failure. www.sign.ac.uk/pdf/sign95.pdf

Smallwood A (2005) Nurse-led elective cardioversion: an evidence based practice review. *Nursing in Critical Care* **10**(5): 231-41.

Stewart S, MacIntyre K, Capewell S and McMurray JJV (2003) Heart failure and the aging population: an increasing burden in the 21st century? *Heart* **89**: 49-53.

Stewart S, Murphy N, McGuire A and McMurray JJV (2002) The current cost of angina pectoris to the National Health Service in the United Kingdom. *Heart* **89**: 848-53.

Thompson D (2007) Improving end-of-life care for patients with chronic heart failure. *Heart* **93**: 901-6.

Vaccarino V, Kasl SV, Abrahamson J *et al.* (2001) Depressive symtoms and risk of functional decline and death in patients with heart failure. *Journal of the American College of Cardiology* **39**(5): 919-21.

Wyse DG, Waldo AL, DiMarco JP *et al.* for AFFIRM Investigators (2002) Atrial fibrillation follow up investigation of rhythm management. *New England Journal of Medicine* **347**: 1825-33.

Zigmond AS and Snaith RP (1983) The hospital anxiety and depression scale. *Acta Psychiatrica Scandinavica* **67**: 361-70.

Web resources

www.cardiomyopathy.org

Chapter 13
Cardiac Rehabilitation

Tim Grove

Introduction

Coronary heart disease (CHD) accounts for the largest proportion of death and disability in industrialised countries (WHO, 2007). The management of these patients is crucial and every healthcare practitioner involved in the care of patients with CHD should actively promote cardiac rehabilitation (CR). CR is a multidisciplinary approach, which aims to improve recovery, enhance long-term adherence to lifestyle changes and promote secondary prevention strategies in patients with CHD (NICE, 2007; SIGN, 2002). Furthermore, it is also a process by which CHD patients are restored to and maintained in the optimal physical and psychosocial function (NICE, 2007; SIGN, 2002). CR begins as soon as the patient arrives in the hospital environment and is ongoing, potentially for the rest of the person's life, in terms of lifestyle changes. Therefore, this chapter and Chapter 14 will focus initially on the hospital phase and move on to the ongoing rehabilitation, which continues in the community setting.

Learning outcomes

At the end of this chapter the reader will be able to:

- describe the phases of cardiac rehabilitation
- discuss the importance of physical activity in a cardiac rehabilitation population
- assess and describe the appropriate interventions for risk factor reduction.

Nursing the Cardiac Patient, First Edition. Edited by Melanie Humphreys.
© 2011 Blackwell Publishing Ltd. Published 2011 by Blackwell Publishing Ltd.

Cardiac rehabilitation in perspective

In the UK there are around 374 CR programmes (NACR, 2008), which vary from centre to centre, but usually include:

- risk factor modification
- supervised exercise sessions
- education and counselling.

To maintain high standards of care several nationally based guidelines have been produced to support CR in the secondary prevention of CHD. The National Service Framework (NSF) for CHD, published in 2000 (DH, 2000), was one of the first and it contains a chapter dedicated to CR. One of the main milestones of the NSF for CHD was that by 2005, 85% of eligible patients discharged from hospital with a primary diagnosis of myocardial infarction (MI) or after coronary revascularisation should be offered CR. However, this milestone is far from being achieved. A recent CR audit in the UK, has demonstrated that only about 47% of cardiac patients are recruited to CR programmes (NACR, 2008).

Since the publication of the NFS, the British Association for Cardiac Rehabilitation (BACR) and the National Institute for Health and Clinical Excellence (NICE) have published up-to-date standards to help promote CR (BACR, 2007; NICE, 2007). The BACR in particular has identified several core components that should be delivered during the four phases of CR. Such components include:

- lifestyle advice
- education
- risk factor management
- psychosocial advice
- cardioprotective drug therapy
- long-term management strategies.

Provision of cardiac rehabilitation

Cardiac rehabilitation in the UK is organised into a four-phased programme (known as phase I, II, III and IV), which aims to restore the cardiac patient to optimal physical and psychosocial function as soon as possible (Figure 13.1). The preliminary phases of CR, phases I to III, are generally led by a multidisciplinary team, which is usually co-ordinated by a cardiac specialist nurse or physiotherapist. Other team members include:

- cardiologists or doctors
- coronary care nurses
- exercise professionals

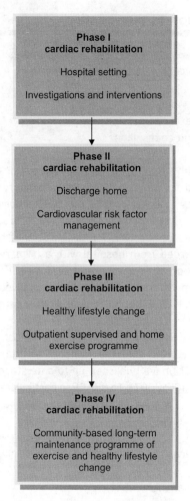

Figure 13.1 Cardiac rehabilitation pathway.

- psychologists
- councillors
- pharmacists
- dieticians
- occupational therapists
- social workers
- physiotherapists.

The level of involvement of each member of the multidisciplinary team varies, but in general the medical practitioners prescribe cardioprotective medication and the allied health professionals empower lifestyle and behaviour change through education and counselling, along with providing a suitable environment in which to exercise. Once these behaviours have been addressed and the patient is medically stable, the usual path of care is a referral to a long-term community-based phase IV CR programme, which is usually led by an exercise professional (BACR, 2006).

Phase I cardiac rehabilitation

Phase I should start immediately after the patient has been admitted to the hospital following an acute coronary syndrome (ST segment elevation MI or non-ST segment elevation MI), or a step change in their cardiac condition, e.g. known angina requiring revascularisation, or an exacerbation in their condition, e.g. heart failure (BACR, 2006). The hospital setting is usually a coronary care unit, medical ward, tertiary centre or a cardiothoracic centre. All patients are eligible for phase I CR. The first component of phase I CR includes an assessment of the patient's physical, psychological and social needs. Relevant information is usually given verbally or written in the form of a booklet on the following areas (BACR, 2006):

- diagnosis and treatment
- risk factor modification
- lifestyle modification
- medication
- management of chest pain and shortness of breath
- physical activity
- anxiety and depression
- returning home, work and travel.

The length of stay in hospital varies from hospital to hospital but generally patients are discharged between two and five days after admission, depending on their condition. The time frames to achieve all the above objectives are limited by the short stay in hospital and they are usually continued into phase II.

Phase II cardiac rehabilitation

Phase II CR takes place in an outpatient setting following discharge from hospital. The care of the patient is transferred back to the GP and CR is usually delivered by the primary care trust or the referring hospital. Phase II lasts between two and six weeks, but is dependent on local provision and the patient's cardiac condition. During phase II the patient should be continually assessed in the following areas (DH, 2000):

- cardiac risk
- physical, psychological and social needs for CR
- provision of lifestyle advice and psychological interventions
- provision of resuscitation training to family members.

The above objectives are normally achieved through follow-up phone calls, risk factor management clinics and home visits. Phase II can be a worrying time for many patients and their family members, as they may feel vulnerable after discharge from hospital. However, phase II is paramount to enhance risk factor and lifestyle changes. Many CR programmes enrol the patient in the Heart Manual, Angioplasty Plan or Angina Plan; these are home-based self-supervised programmes with medical support (Lewin *et al.*, 1992, 2002). These programmes can be used as a sole CR programme or in conjunction with a formal CR programme. The beneficial effects of home-based CR are comparable to centre-based CR. This has been demonstrated in a recent meta-analysis, which showed that home- and centre-based forms of CR are equally effective in reducing mortality and cardiac events, risk factor reduction and improving health-related quality of life in patients following an MI or revascularisation (Dalal *et al.*, 2010).

During phase II, patients may also be invited to attend educational talks on various topics such as:

- CHD
- medication
- diet
- physical activity
- stress management
- relaxation techniques.

Phase III cardiac rehabilitation

Phase III CR can start at any time and is usually dependent on local provision and the cardiac status of the patient. In general, patients start phase III two weeks following planned percutaneous coronary intervention, four to six weeks post uncomplicated MI and six to eight weeks post cardiac surgery (BACR, 2006). During phase III, patients start a formal rehabilitation programme with individualised and group exercise sessions.

The first step in the assessment of the patient during phase III includes a clinical history, the results of any investigations to rule out contra-indications to exercise (coronary angiography, echocardiograms, stress ECG, etc.), a physical examination (resting heart rate, blood pressure, body mass index and waist circumference), and physical and psychological tests. Physical tests usually take the form of an exercise test, which might include a treadmill test, incremental shuttle walk test (Singh *et al.*, 1992), Chester step test (Sykes, 2003) or the six-minute walk test (Butland *et al.*, 1982). The purpose of these tests is to help determine functional capacity, risk stratification, to set appropriate exercise intensities and to measure the effects of the CR programme. Furthermore, simple psychological tests can be used to measure depression and quality of life before and after the programme. Such psychological tests include the hospital anxiety and depression scale (Zigmond and Snaith, 1983) and Short-Form 36 (SF-36v2) functional limitation questionnaire (Ware and Sherbourne, 1992).

Following the assessment, a medically based supervised exercise programme and home programme can be started. The benefits of regular exercise in lowering total and cardiac mortality in patients with established CHD have been well documented (Clarke *et al.*, 2005; Taylor *et al.*, 2004). A recent meta-analysis of 8,940 men and women showed that exercise-based CR programmes reduce all cause mortality by 27% and cardiac mortality by 31% compared with patients receiving usual care (Taylor *et al.*, 2004). These findings have been echoed in a much larger meta-analysis of 21,295 patients, which showed that secondary prevention programmes, including risk factor counselling or education along with regular exercise sessions, reduced mortality and recurrent MI rates (Clarke *et al.*, 2005). This meta-analysis demonstrated that CR programmes with exercise had a non-significant 12% effect on reducing mortality and a significant 38% positive effect on reducing recurrent MIs. Furthermore, CR programmes without exercise had a 23% positive effect on lowering mortality (which was significant) and a non-significant 14% benefit on reducing recurrent MIs.

Phase IV cardiac rehabilitation

Phase IV CR usually follows phase III and is normally delivered in the community. The community setting is the preferred choice as it promotes independence. The purpose of phase IV is to promote the long-term maintenance of health behaviours that were achieved during phases I, II and III. Phase IV is usually led by a BACR exercise instructor and involves the patient attending regular exercise sessions, which are similar in nature to the exercise class in the phase III setting. The limited number of studies that have investigated the long-term benefits of phase IV CR have shown that it continues to improve quality of life, promotes smoking cessation adherence and offers social support (Willmer and Waite 2009; Thow *et al.*, 2008).

Summary

Every healthcare professional involved in the care of patients with CHD should actively promote cardiac rehabilitation. Rehabilitation consists of four phases, which aim to promote lifestyle advice, education, risk factor management, psychosocial advice, nutrition advice, cardioprotective drug therapy, supervised exercise sessions and long-term management strategies. CR has been shown to reduce total and cardiac mortality when compared with usual care. However, the uptake of this specific and focused rehabilitation is low and each aspect of the rehabilitation pathway should take into account social, cultural and financial considerations, and all lifestyle inventions must be tailored to the individual.

References

British Association for Cardiac Rehabilitation (BACR) (2007) *Standards and Core Components for Cardiac Rehabilitation*. Available at www.bcs.com/documents/affiliates/bacr/BACR%20Standards%202007.pdf (accessed July 2008).

British Association for Cardiac Rehabilitation (BACR) (2006) *BACR Phase IV Training Module Manual* (4e). Leeds, Human Kinetics.

Butland RJ, Pang J, Gross ER *et al.* (1982) Two-, six-, and twelve-minute walking tests in respiratory disease. *British Medical Journal* **284**: 1607-8.

Clarke AM, Harting L, Vandermeer B *et al.* (2005) Meta-analysis: secondary prevention programmes for patients with coronary artery disease. *Annals of Internal Medicine* **143**(9): 659-72.

Dalal HM, Zawada A, Jolly K, Moxham T and Taylor RS (2010) Home based versus centre based cardiac rehabiltiation: Cochrane systematic review and meta-analysis. *British Medical Journal* **2010**: 340.

Department of Health (2000) *National Service Framework for Coronary Heart Disease*. London, Department of Health.

Lewin RJP, Furze G, Robinson J *et al.* (2002) A randomised controlled trial of a self-management plan for patients with newly diagnosed angina. *British Journal of General Practice* **52**: 194-201.

Lewin RJP, Robertson IH, Cay EL *et al.* (1992) A self-help post-MI rehabilitation package – The Heart Manual: effects on psychological adjustment, hospitalisation and GP consultation. *Lancet* **339**: 1036-40.

National Audit of Cardiac Rehabilitation (NACR) (2008) *Annual Statistical Report 2008*. British Heart Foundation. Available at www.cardiacrehabilitation.org.uk/dataset.htm (accessed June 2009).

National Institute for Health and Clinical Excellence (NICE) (2007) *MI: Secondary Prevention in Primary and Secondary Care for Patients following a Myocardial Infarction*. NICE Clinical Guideline 48. Available at www.nice.org.uk/nicemedia/pdf/CG48NICEGuidance.pdf (accessed July 2008).

Scottish Intercollegiate Guidelines Network (SIGN) (2000) *Cardiac Rehabilitation, no. 57*. Edinburgh, SIGN.

Singh SJ, Morgan MD, Scott S *et al.* (1992) Development of a shuttle walking test of disability in patients with chronic airways obstruction. *Thorax* **47**: 1019-24.

Sykes K (2003) *The Chester Step Test*. Wrexham, Assist Publications.

Taylor RS, Brown A, Ebrahim S *et al.* (2004) Exercise-based rehabilitation for patients with coronary heart disease: systematic review and meta-analysis of randomized controlled trials. *American Journal of Medicine* **116**: 682-92.

Thow M, Rafferty D and Kelly H (2008) Exercise motives of long-term phase IV cardiac rehabilitation participants. *Physiotherapy* **94**(4): 281-5.

Ware JE and Sherbourne CD (1992) The MOS 36-item short-form health survey (SF 36), I: conceptual framework and item selection. *Medical Care* **30**: 473-83.

Willmer KA and Waite M (2009) Long-term benefits of cardiac rehabilitation: a five-year follow-up of community-based phase 4 programmes. *British Journal of Cardiology* **16**: 73-7.

World Health Organization (WHO) (2007) *Cardiovascular Diseases Fact Sheet*. Available at www.who.int/mediacentre/factsheets/fs317/en/index.html (accessed June 2009).

Zigmond AS and Snaith RP (1983) The hospital anxiety and depression scale. *Acta Psychiatrica Scandinavica* **67**: 361-70.

Chapter 14

Secondary Prevention Within the Community

Tim Grove

Introduction

Secondary prevention continues in the community setting for all cardiac patients. It goes on with a multidisciplinary focus which aims to maintain the recovery process, enhance long-term adherence to lifestyle changes and promote concordance with secondary prevention strategies in patients with coronary heart disease (CHD) (BACR, 2007; NICE, 2007; SIGN, 2000). It is extremely important once the patient has been discharged to ensure that optimal physical and psychosocial functions are maintained. This chapter develops on Chapter 13, focusing on those aspects of cardiac rehabilitation (CR) that may well have been commenced during the inpatient phase. CR will be continued to promote optimal recovery and potentially influence the rest of the person's life, certainly in terms of lifestyle changes.

Learning outcomes

At the end of this chapter the reader will be able to:

- describe the important elements within long-term management of the cardiac patient
- discuss the continued importance of physical activity in a cardiac rehabilitation population
- assess and describe the appropriate interventions for ongoing risk factor reduction.

Since the publication of the National Service Framework for Coronary Heart Disease (DH, 2000), the British Association for Cardiac Rehabilitation (BACR) and the National Institute for Health and Clinical Excellence (NICE) have

Nursing the Cardiac Patient, First Edition. Edited by Melanie Humphreys.
© 2011 Blackwell Publishing Ltd. Published 2011 by Blackwell Publishing Ltd.

published up-to-date standards to help promote CR (BACR, 2007; NICE, 2007). The BACR in particular has identified several core components that should be delivered during the four phases of CR – these phases are discussed in Chapter 13. Such components include:

- lifestyle advice
- education
- risk factor management
- psychosocial advice
- cardioprotective drug therapy
- long-term management strategies.

While many of these initiatives commence in the inpatient setting, many will continue in the community, particularly those aimed at long-term management.

Ongoing risk factor modification

Most of the present literature discusses CR in terms of the exercise component and sometimes fails to mention the importance of ongoing risk factor modification. Risk factor education or counselling without exercise is associated with a significant 23% positive effect on lowering total mortality and 14% non-significant reduction in recurrent myocardial infarction (MI) respectively (Clarke et al., 2005). Therefore modifiable risk factors should be aggressively managed to meet the recommendations through smoking cessation counselling, diet and cardioprotective medication (Box 14.1).

Smoking cessation

Patients should be encouraged to stop smoking as soon as possible, normally in phase I CR. To support the cessation of smoking, UK guidelines propose that every health professional involved in CR use the "five As" (Aveyard and West, 2007).

- Ask about smoking history.
- Advise patients to stop.
- Assess motivation to stop and the need for pharmacotherapy.
- Assist with prescription or referral to a behavioural support programme.
- Arrange a follow-up.

Cardiac nurses play a vital role in encouraging patients to abstain from smoking. Research has shown that 57% of cardiac patients admitted to hospital with an MI, unstable angina or who have undergone bypass surgery will quit smoking following simple advice given by a cardiac nurse (Quist-Paulsen and Gallefoss, 2003).

Box 14.1 Lifestyle recommendations and cardiovascular disease risk factor targets

- Do not smoke
- Limit alcohol intake to <3-4 units for a man per day; <2-3 units for a woman per day
- Keep blood pressure <130/80 mm Hg through medication and or lifestyle advice
- Keep total cholesterol to <4.0 mmol/l and LDL cholesterol <2.0 mmol/l through medication and lifestyle advice
- Control fasting blood glucose to <6 mmol/l and HbA1c <6.5% through medication and/or lifestyle advice
- Maintain ideal bodyweight for adults (body mass index 20 25 kg/m^2) and avoid central obesity (waist circumference in white Caucasians <102 cm in men and <88 cm in women, and in Asians <90 cm in men and <80 cm in women)
- In overweight and obese patients an initial weight loss should be set at 5-10% of total bodyweight
- Follow a Mediterranean-style diet, keeping total dietary intake of fat to <30% of total energy intake, with total saturated fat kept to <10% of total fat in take
- Increase the intake of oily fish and other sources of omega-3 fatty acids (at least two to three servings of oily fish per week)
- Keep the intake of dietary cholesterol <300 mg/day
- Reduce salt intake to <100 mmol/l day (<6 g of sodium chloride or <2.4 g of sodium per day)
- Increase aerobic physical activity to at least 30 minutes per day, performed on five or more days of the week (for example brisk walking, cycling, cardiac rehabilitation exercise classes, home exercise programme)

Adapted from Wood et al., (2005)

Diet and CHD

Healthy eating is one of the cornerstones in the treatment of CHD and other associated risk factors such as high cholesterol, hypertension, diabetes and obesity. Current dietetic guidelines for secondary prevention of cardiovascular disease recommend the following (Mead et al., 2006).

- Advice on the Mediterranean diet.
- Increased omega-3 fat intake from dietary or supplemental fish oils.
- A reduction in saturated fats and total or partial replacement by unsaturated fats.

Table 14.1 Dietary items included in the original Mediterranean diet questionnaire

Dietary item	Yes	No
1. Olive oil (>1 tablespoon/day)	+1	0
2. Fruit (>1 serving/day)	+1	0
3. Vegetables or salad (>1 serving/day)	+1	0
4. Fruit (>1 serving/day) and vegetable (>1 serving/day)[a]	+1	0
5. Legumes (>2 serving/week)	+1	0
6. Fish (>3 serving/week)	+1	0
7. Wine (>1 glass/day, 3-4 units/day male and 2-3 units/day female)	+1	0
8. Meat (<1 serving/day pork, beef or lamb)	+1	0
9. White bread (<1 serving/day) and rice (<1 serving/ week) or wholegrain bread (>5 serving/week)[b]	+1	0

[a]One point should be added when 3 servings/day of fruit and 2 servings/day of vegetables are consumed.
[b]One point is added when either consumption of both white bread and rice is low or when consumption of whole grain bread is high.
Adapted with permission from Martínez-González et al., 2004.

In practice, the Mediterranean diet can be accessed through the Mediterranean diet scale, which consists of a questionnaire covering nine components (Table 14.1). The components of the questionnaire are scored on the amount of fish, nuts, alcohol, vegetables and fruit consumed on a daily or a weekly basis. The nine components are assigned the values of 0 or 1, depending on the level of consumption. For instance 0 is assigned to a person whose consumption of beneficial components (vegetables, fruits, fish, etc.) is below the recommended amounts, whereas the value of 1 is assigned to a person who meets the recommended beneficial amounts. The Mediterranean score represents the adherence to the diet and can be scored as poor adherence (score 0-2), average adherence (score of 5-6) and very good adherence (score of >7) (Trichopoulou et al., 2005). A recent observational study has shown that a two-unit increase in the Mediterranean score was associated with a 27% and a 31% lower total mortality rate and a lower cardiac mortality rate among persons with CHD respectively (Trichopoulou et al., 2005).

Since the development of the original Mediterranean scale, Estruch et al. (2006) have developed a more detailed scale covering 14 components of the Mediterranean diet (Table 14.2). This scale might be more appealing for health professionals to use in practice when assessing the dietary needs of their patients.

Table 14.2 Quantitative score of adherence to the Mediterranean diet

Foods and frequency of consumption	Criteria for 1 point*
1. Do you use olive oil as main culinary fat?	Yes
2. How much olive oil do you consume in a given day (including oil used for frying, salads, out-of-house meals, etc.)?	>4 tablespoons
3. How many vegetable servings do you consume per day? (1 serving = 200 g [consider side dishes as half a serving])	>2 (>1 portion raw or as salad)
4. How many fruit units (including natural fruit juices) do you consume per day?	>3
5. How many servings of red meat, hamburger or meat products (ham, sausage, etc.) do you consume per day? (1 serving = 100-150 g)	<1
6. How many servings of butter, margarine or cream do you consume per day? (1 serving = 12 g)	<1
7. How many sweet or carbonated beverages do you drink per day?	<1
8. How much wine do you drink per week?	>3 glasses
9. How many servings of legumes do you consume per week? (1 serving = 150 g)	>3
10. How many servings of fish or shellfish do you consume per week? (1 serving = 100-150 g of fish or 4-5 units or 200 g of shellfish)	>3
11. How many times per week do you consume commercial sweets or pastries (not homemade), such as cakes, cookies, biscuits, or custard?	<3
12. How many servings of nuts (including peanuts) do you consume per week? (1 serving = 30 g)	>1
13. Do you preferentially consume chicken, turkey or rabbit meat instead of veal, pork, hamburger, or sausage?	Yes
14. How many times per week do you consume vegetables, pasta, rice or other dishes seasoned with *sofrito* (sauce made with tomato and onion, leek, or garlic and simmered with olive oil)?	>2

*0 points if these criteria are not met.
Adapted with permission from Estruch *et al.*, 2006.

Omega-3 fatty acids

One of the major components of the Mediterranean diet is an increase in the consumption of oily fish, which contains omega-3 fatty acids, examples of which are salmon, mackerel, herring and fresh tuna. Omega-3 fatty acids have been shown to reduce platelet aggregation, arrhythmias, very-low-density lipoproteins, triglycerides and the risk of developing heart failure (Truswell, 2003; Levitan *et al.*, 2009).

Fat intake

Dietary fat is one of the major sources of energy and there four types of fat consumed in the diet:

- monounsaturated fat
- polyunsaturated fat
- saturated fat
- trans fat.

Dietetic guidelines recommend that total fat intake should be kept below 30% of total energy intake in CHD patients (Mead *et al.*, 2006). In addition, saturated fat should be kept below 10% of total fat intake and should partially be replaced by monounsaturated or polyunsaturated fat (Mead *et al.*, 2006).

Diet and blood pressure

In the context of the current recommendations, a diet rich in fruits and vegetables and low in salt and saturated fat has a significant impact on lowering blood pressure (BP). This has been demonstrated in two large, highly acclaimed multi-centre randomised controlled trials known as the Dietary Approaches to Stop Hypertension (DASH) (Sacks *et al.*, 2001; Appel *et al.*, 1997). Both trials had a sample size of more than 400 subjects who had normal BP or were classified as hypertensive. The results of the first trial showed that a diet rich in fruits, vegetables, low-fat dairy foods, whole grains, seeds and nuts reduced BP in normotensive and hypertensive subjects by 5.5mmHg and 3.0mmHg (systolic and diastolic) and 11.4mmHg and 3.0mmHg respectively (Appel *et al.*, 1997). In the second trial, the same dietary intervention was followed, with the addition of a restriction in sodium. The second trial showed a further reduction in systolic BP in normotensive and hypertensive subjects by 7.1mmHg and 11.5mmHg respectively (Sacks *et al.*, 2001). A reduction in BP by an average 12/6mmHg can be expected to reduce the risk of CHD by 20% (Wood *et al.*, 2005).

Diet and cholesterol

Elevated blood cholesterol concentrations, especially low-density lipoproteins (LDL) are one of the key risk factors for the development of CHD.

Dietary interventions should aim to reduce LDL cholesterol while at the same time maintaining or increasing high-density lipoproteins (HDL). Diets that are high in monounsaturated fats and low in saturated fat, for example the Mediterranean diet, has been shown to have a beneficial effect on lowering LDL cholesterol and increasing HDL cholesterol when compared with low fat diets (Estruch et al., 2006; Mensink et al., 2003).

Diet and diabetes

Diabetes is a complex condition that requires intensive management through lifestyle change and medication. Dietary interventions form the main component for the treatment of patients with diabetes. There are many types of diabetes, with type II diabetes being the most prevalent in a CR population. The exact dietary interventions for patients with diabetes are beyond the scope of this chapter; however, research into the effects of the Mediterranean diet on glycaemic control have been promising (Estruch et al., 2006).

Diet and weight management

It is vital that patients with established CHD achieve or maintain a body mass index (BMI) of <25 kg/m^2 and achieve or maintain a waist circumference of <102 cm for men and <88 cm for women However, weight loss for some patients is very challenging and they may require intensive behavioural therapy to achieve their ideal body weight. Generally, patients with a BMI greater than 30 kg/m^2 should be referred to a dietician, although these services are not always available to all CR programmes.

However, simple advice following the recommendations outlined in Box 14.1 along with regular exercise may provoke a change in body weight. Weight reduction should be achieved through negative energy balance. However, essential nutrients should not be compromised and the goal is to reduce body fat and increase or preserve lean body mass. Food habits can be identified through food diaries and food frequency questionnaires, which can be analysed and recommendations given based on the findings. Overweight and obese patients should initially aim to lose about 10% of their body weight. A 10% weight reduction has been associated with a 20% reduction in total mortality, 10% reduction in total cholesterol and 10 mmHg and 20 mmHg reduction in systolic and diastolic blood pressure respectively (Logue et al., 2010).

Psychological wellbeing

When an individual encounters a life-threatening event such as an MI they will normally experience some form of psychological emotion. Psychological emotions cover a wide spectrum of feelings, which might include anger, hostility, denial, bargaining, anxiety and depression. Anger and hostility are fairly common emotions after a cardiac event as some patients feel that a particular event such as stress has caused their heart attack. However, patients might present with anger and hostility pre-cardiac event, which is a part of their normal behaviour pattern. Such patients are classified as having a type A personality, which increases their risk of CHD (Stansfeld and Marmot, 2002).

Denial and bargaining

Denial and bargaining are also common in patients following a cardiac event. Denial can be seen as a coping mechanism to help elevate any fears or anxiety in well-informed patients. However, denial can also be counter-productive in promoting unhealthy lifestyle behaviours and poor medical compliance.

Anxiety

Anxiety is very common following a cardiac event and is characterised as a state of apprehension, tension and worry, which can manifest into physical symptoms such as:

- rapid heart rate
- increased respiration rate
- pins and needles
- shaking or trembling
- stomach churning
- heart palpitations
- dizziness.

Patterns of anxiety vary throughout the time course of recovery in patients with CHD. For instance, anxiety declines during hospital stay when the patient's clinical condition has stabilised and then might rise following discharge home (Brodie, 2000). Anxiety has been associated with an increased risk of developing depression if left untreated (Lichtman et al., 2008).

Depression

Depression and depressive symptoms are a mood disorder, which features extreme dejection, melancholy, lack of motivation, and feelings of hopelessness and low self-esteem (Brodie, 2000; BACR, 1995). In addition, some patients experience physical symptoms such as chronic fatigue, loss of appetite and disturbed sleep (Brodie, 2000; BACR, 1995). The prevalence of depression following a cardiac event has been estimated to range between 15 and 20% (Milani et al., 1996; Schleifer et al., 1989; Carney et al., 1987), and left untreated, depressive symptoms will remain for up to one year or more. However, many of these patients might have been depressed pre-cardiac event (Glassman et al., 2006).

Depression following a recent cardiac event such an MI is associated with a two- to fourfold increase in cardiac and all-cause mortality (Milani and Lavie, 2007; van Melle *et al.*, 2004), poor quality of life (Lichtman *et al.*, 2008) and increased healthcare costs (Frasure-Smith *et al.*, 2000). The potential mechanisms linking depression with a poor cardiac prognosis are not fully understood. However, several factors, such as increased sympathetic nervous system activity (resulting in fatal arrhythmic events) and the adoption of unhealthy lifestyle behaviours (unhealthy eating, inactivity and tobacco use), have been documented as a plausible explanation linking depression with a poor cardiac prognosis (Kronish *et al.*, 2006; Carney *et al.*, 1993). Furthermore, depression has also been linked to non-compliance of medical treatment regimens, medication and poor adherence to CR (Lichtman *et al.*, 2008). Therefore, it would be prudent to assess and treat depressive illness first in CHD patients before implementing any of the health behaviour changes.

Assessment of psychological factors

The true diagnosis of depression should be determined after a structured interview carried out by a health professional who specialises in mental health. However, mental health professionals such as clinical psychologists are not always available to CR services (NACR, 2008). Therefore CHD patients should be screened by the CR team for the probability of depression at discharge with the process repeated at 6–12 weeks post event and then repeated at three-monthly intervals (SIGN, 2000). This will help tailor treatment.

To help screen for depression there are several assessment tools in the format of questionnaires that are used to evaluate psychosocial issues in CHD patients. These questionnaires include the hospital anxiety and depression scale (Zigmond and Snaith, 1983), the general health questionnaire (Vieweg and Hedlund, 1983) and the Beck depression inventory (Beck *et al.*, 1961). These questionnaires are easy to score and can help identity patients at high risk of depression who might benefit from several treatment options.

Psychosocial treatments

There are several evidence-based treatments that can be offered to CHD patients with depression. Options include cognitive behavioural therapy (CBT), medication and exercise-based CR. These treatments should be offered in discussion with the patient and, where appropriate, a family member.

Cognitive behavioural therapy

CBT targets the beliefs, motivations and environmental factors that influence the patient's unwanted behaviours and involves the patient systematically practising alternative behaviours (Brodie, 2000). CBT is usually delivered by a clinical psychologist, although other healthcare professionals trained in CBT can offer effective treatment. The benefits of CBT have been shown to achieve remission in patients with moderate to severe depression after 12 to 16 sessions over a 12-week period (Lichtman et al., 2008). Other psychological treatments such as motivational interviewing, stress management and relaxation techniques have also been shown to be effective treatments for depression (SIGN, 2002). The overall benefits of psychological treatments have been demonstrated in a recent meta-analysis (Linden et al., 2007), which concluded that such treatments reduced mortality and event recurrence in cardiac patients by 27% and 43% respectively over a two-year period.

Antidepressant drugs

There are three main classes of drugs used to treat depression: tricyclics, selective serotonin re-uptake inhibitors (SSRIs) and the monoamine oxidase inhibitors. However, SSRIs are one of the only forms of antidepressant drug that are safe to use in CHD patients (NICE, 2007b; Davies et al., 2004). There are two main types of SSRIs, sertraline and citalopram. These two drugs have been shown to reduce death or recurrent MI by 42% in CHD patients with moderate to severe depression (Lichtman et al., 2008).

Cardiac rehabilitation

Exercise-based CR has shown positive effects on reducing depressive symptoms with subsequent reductions in mortality in CHD patients (Milani and Lavie, 2007). This has been demonstrated in a recent non-randomised clinical trial, which showed that CR decreased the prevalence of depressive symptoms by 63% and mortality by 73% (Milani and Lavie, 2007). The improvements in depressive symptoms following CR are likely to be multifactorial. As discussed earlier in the chapter, CR offers education and counselling along with exercise, which may all play key roles in reducing depressive symptoms. Furthermore, the group element of CR might offer social support, which may reduce depressive symptoms.

Exercise prescription

Physical activity and structured exercise programmes significantly improve the health outcomes in patients with CHD. Generally, most CR programmes offer between one and two supervised exercise sessions a week, which is supplemented with a home exercise programme. The prescription of exercise is normally delivered by an appropriately trained exercise professional or physiotherapist. The exercise prescription is devised using the FITT principle, which stands for frequency, intensity, time and type, and it is described later in this section.

When prescribing exercise it is important that all cardiac patients undergo a graduated warm-up for 15 minutes. This serves to gradually dilate the coronary arteries, whereupon the anginal/ischaemic threshold will be prolonged and the chance of arrhythmias will be reduced (ACSM 2005; BACR, 1995,

2006). A similar process lasting 10 minutes should be performed at the end of an exercise session, which acts as the cool-down period. During this time stretching can be performed.

Frequency: the health benefits related to physical activity follow a dose-response relationship. For instance, some physical activity is better than none, but greater amounts will bestow greater benefit. Therefore, the frequency of exercise should follow public health messages, which recommends that most adults should perform at least 30 minutes of moderate intensity physical activity on at least five days of the week (DH, 2004).

Intensity: exercise intensity is usually set using heart rate response and the patient's ratings of perceived exertion (RPE). The optimal exercise intensity should be set at 60–80% of the maximal heart rate response achieved during a symptom-limited exercise test or it can be calculated from the age predicted maximal heart rate (e.g. 220 minus age multiplied by 0.60 or 0.80). However, it should be noted that heart rate response might be limited in some patients who have a history of diabetes, heart failure or are taking beta blockade therapy. Therefore exercise intensity can be guided using the Borg RPE scale (Borg, 1998). The Borg RPE scale is a 6–20 scale, which asks the participant to rate their perceived level of exertion during exercise. The number 6 on the exertion scale represents "no exertion" and 20 represents "maximal exertion" (Borg, 1998). The patient's perception of exercise intensity has been shown to correlate well with heart rate response (Pollock *et al.*, 1991), and it is recommended that the exercise levels be set between 11 and 13, "fairly light" and "somewhat hard" (BACR, 2006; ACSM, 2005).

Time: the length of time spent during each session is dependent on the patient's cardiovascular fitness level and personal goals. Generally most CR exercise classes last one hour (15 minutes warm up, 20–30 minutes circuit interval training and 10 minutes cool-down). However, patients with low fitness levels might require shorter bouts of exercise, which can be performed several times throughout the day (e.g. three bouts of 10 minutes). Benefits of regular exercise training include:

- CAD suppression and regression (Hambrecht *et al.*, 1994)
- lower ratio of total to high-density lipoprotein cholesterol (Ades *et al.*, 2009)
- lower triglyceride cholesterol levels (Ades *et al.*, 2009)
- reduced insulin resistance (Ades *et al.*, 2009)
- educed blood pressure (Ades *et al.*, 2009).

Other benefits of regular exercise are summarised in Figure 14.1.

Type: supervised CR exercise sessions usually consist of aerobic and muscular strength endurance training, which are normally alternated as part of a circuit class (Appendix A shows a typical CR exercise circuit). It should be noted that patients attending exercise-based CR should not present with any

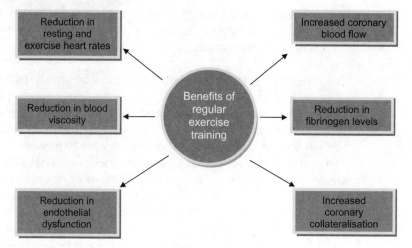

Figure 14.1 Benefits of regular exercise training.

Box 14.2 Absolute contraindications to exercise (based on the BACR 2006 contraindications to exercise)

- Fever and acute systemic illness
- Unstable angina
- Exertional angina at low levels of exercise
- Resting BP systolic >180 mm Hg or diastolic >100 mm Hg
- Significant unexplained drop in BP during exercise
- Tachycardia >100 bpm
- New or recurrent symptoms of breathlessness, palpitations, dizziness or lethargy
- Unstable diabetes
- Unstable heart failure

---

of the contra-indications to exercise and they should be risk stratified to predict cardiovascular events during exercise (Boxes 14.2 and 14.3).

Home-based exercise programme

As discussed earlier, most CR programmes only offer between one-to-two supervised exercise sessions per week. Therefore, it is important for the patient to participate in a home based exercise programme to achieve the desired "dose" of exercise, which is at least 30 minutes of moderate intensity aerobic exercise performed on five days of the week (DH, 2004). To achieve this goal, walking is one of the easiest ways to exercise, it requires no skill or equipment, and it is socially acceptable with no age, gender or race

Box 14.3 AACVPR Stratification of risk for cardiac events during exercise participation

Characteristics of patients at lowest risk for exercise participation

All characteristics must be present for patient to remain at the lowest risk.

- Absence of complex ventricular arrhythmias during exercise testing and recovery.
- Absence of angina or other significant symptoms (e.g. unusual shortness of breath, light headedness or dizziness during exercise testing and recovery).
- Presence of normal haemodynamics during exercise testing and recovery (i.e. appropriate increases and decreases in heart rate and systolic blood pressure with increasing workloads and recovery).
- Functional capacity >7 metabolic equivalents of activity (METs).

Non-exercise testing findings:

- rest ejection fraction >50%
- uncomplicated MI or revascularisation procedure
- absence of complicated ventricular arrhythmias at rest
- absence of CHF
- absence of signs and symptoms of post event/post procedure ischaemia
- absence of clinical depression.

Characteristics of patients at moderate risk for exercise participation

Any one or combination of these findings places the person at moderate risk.

- Presence of angina or other significant symptoms (e.g. shortness of breath, light headedness, or dizziness occurring at high levels of exertion (>7 METs).
- Mild to moderate level of silent ischaemia during exercise testing or recovery (ST-segment depression <2 mm from baseline).
- Functional capacity <5 MET.

Non-exercise testing findings:

- rest ejection fraction = 40–49%.

(Continued)

> ### Box 14.3 (Continued)
>
> **Characteristics of patients at high risk for exercise participation**
>
> Any one or combination of these findings places the person at high risk.
>
> - Presence of complex ventricular arrhythmias during exercise testing and recovery.
> - Presence of angina or other significant symptoms (e.g. shortness of breath, light headedness or dizziness occurring at low levels of exertion (<5 METs) or during recovery.
> - High level of silent ischaemia (ST segment depression >2 mm from baseline) during exercise testing or recovery.
> - Presence of abnormal haemodynamics during exercise testing (i.e. chronotropic incompetence or flat or decreasing systolic BP with increasing workloads) or recovery (i.e. severe post-exercise hypotension).
>
> Non-exercise testing findings:
>
> - rest ejection fraction <40%
> - history of cardiac arrest, or sudden death
> - complex dysrhythmias at rest
> - complicated MI or revascularisation procedure
> - presence of CHF
> - presence of signs and symptoms of post-event/post-procedure ischaemia
> - presence of clinical depression.
>
> Reprinted from Williams (2004), with permission from Elsevier.

barriers. Walking should be encouraged in most cardiac patients and the health professional should encourage the use of the RPE scale (Borg, 1998) to set the walking pace.

Psychosocial wellbeing

Sexual relationships

Sexual problems related to atherosclerosis, side effects of medical therapies, e.g. beta-blockers, or psychological factors (anxiety and depression) are common in patients with CHD. Therefore it is essential that the patient and partner are happy to discuss their sexual relationships before offering any advice. For those wishing to discuss such matters, advice can be given to help alleviate some of the fears surrounding sexual activity. One scenario might be the fear of provoking cardiovascular complications (angina, dyspnoea and palpitations) during sexual intercourse. This may lead to loss of libido and impotence for both the patient and partner. However, the patient and their partner can be reassured that if symptoms such as angina, dyspnoea or palpitations are absent during moderate exertion physical activity, they are unlikely to occur during sexual intercourse (Kostis et al., 2005). The reader is referred to Kostis et al. (2005) for a more detailed discussion in the area of sexual dysfunction and cardiac risk.

Return to work

There are several limiting factors that might influence the patient's ability to return to work following a cardiac event. Such limitations include low functional capacity, poor prognosis, reduced self-efficacy or inappropriate perceptions of actual job demands (ACSM, 2005). Exercise training may enhance the patient's decision to return to work by improving self-efficacy (ACSM, 2005). In addition, aerobic and resistance training have been shown to improve the physiological (heart rate and blood pressure) response to a given workload, which might be advantageous for patients returning to a manual occupation (ACSM, 2005). The decision on the time frames for when a patient can return to work should be discussed in conjunction with the patient, employer, GP and CR team.

Travel

Travelling long distances should be avoided until the patient is medically stable. Planned travel should be discussed with the CR team, and high altitudes (>1500 m) and extreme temperatures should be avoided (Dickstein et al., 2008). In general, air travel is preferable to long journeys by other means of transportation (Dickstein et al., 2008).

Cardioprotective medication

Drug therapy is an important part of CR secondary prevention programmes. This section discusses in brief the importance of some of the major drug therapies used in secondary prevention; further information can be found in more comprehensive cardiac books. The following recommendations are based on the recent NICE guidelines (NICE, 2007a), which advocate that all patients who have had an acute MI should be offered treatment with a combination of the following drugs:

- ACE (angiotensin-converting enzyme) inhibitor
- aspirin
- beta-blocker
- HMG-CoA reductase inhibitors (statins).

The effects of combination drug therapies in patients with CAD have been well documented. Hippisley-Cox and Coupland (2005) have demonstrated a 70–80% reduction in all-cause mortality with drug therapy combinations including ACE inhibitors, aspirin, beta-blockers and statins.

ACE inhibitors

NICE recommends that ACE inhibitors should be offered to all patients following an acute MI (NICE, 2007a). In the past, ACE inhibitors were used in the treatment of left ventricular dysfunction and heart failure. However, mortality benefits have now been recognised in MI patients with preserved left ventricular function (Yusuf et al., 2000). ACE inhibitor therapy should be started as soon as possible, at an appropriate level and titrated upwards at short intervals until the maximum tolerated or target dose is reached (NICE, 2007a). ACE inhibitor therapy is also one of the first-line treatments for hypertension and should be used to achieve optimal blood pressure control (<130/80 mm Hg). However, if ACE inhibitor therapy is not well tolerated, angiotensin receptor blockers may be recommended as an alternative (NICE, 2007a).

Aspirin

Aspirin should be offered to all patients after an acute MI, and should be continued indefinitely (NICE, 2007a). Generally, aspirin and other anti-platelet therapies are recommended for all patients with established athero-sclerotic disease (Wood et al., 2005). Anti-platelet therapy has been shown in meta-analyses to significantly reduce the risk in all-cause mortality, vascular mortality, non-fatal re-infarction of the myocardium, and non-fatal stroke in unstable angina, acute MI, stroke, transient ischaemic attacks or other evidence of vascular disease (Antithrombotic Trialists' Collaboration, 2002; Antiplatelet Trialists' Collaboration, 1994).

Other anti-platelet therapies include a combination of clopidogrel and low-dose aspirin, which is reserved for high-risk patients who have suffered a non-ST segment elevation MI or have undergone percutaneous coronary interventions (NICE, 2007a). In general, such patients can be offered combination therapy for at least 12 months. In addition, clopidogrel can be offered as an alternative to patients who are intolerant to aspirin (NICE, 2007a).

Beta-blockers

Beta-blockers are used in the treatment of myocardial ischaemia, heart failure and cardiovascular disease protection following an MI, and are also used as a second-line treatment in hypertension (Wood *et al.*, 2005). The benefits of beta-blockers have been well documented in a recent meta-analysis by Freemantle *et al.* (1999), which showed evidence of significant reductions in all-cause mortality, cardiovascular death and in particular sudden cardiac death, as well as non-fatal re-infarction. Beta-blockers should be offered soon after an acute MI when the patient is clinically stable, and continued indefinitely (NICE, 2007a).

HMG-CoA reductase inhibitors

HMG-CoA reductase inhibitors (statin therapy) are hypolipidemic drugs, which are recommended for adults with clinical evidence of cardiovascular disease (NICE, 2007a). Statin therapy has been shown to reduce the relative risk of death by 30% (Scandinavian Simvastatin Survival Study Group, 1994) and should be the first-line treatment for reducing total and LDL cholesterol (NICE, 2007a). These findings have been supported by a meta-analysis of statin trials, which comprised of more than 90,000 patients (Baigent *et al.*, 2005). In this meta-analysis a reduction of 1mmol/l in LDL cholesterol resulted in a 12% proportional reduction in all-cause mortality, a 19% reduction in coronary mortality and a 24% reduction in the need for coronary revascularisation (Baigent *et al.*, 2005). Statin therapy should be offered as soon as possible following a cardiovascular event regardless of the initial cholesterol value (NICE, 2007a). This has been supported by three clinical trials, which have assessed the short-term impact of the immediate use of statin therapy. The three trials concluded that early statin therapy reduces early mortality following an acute coronary syndrome (Cannon *et al.*, 2004; de Lemos *et al.*, 2004; Schwartz *et al.*, 2001). Statin therapy should be continued indefinitely and gradually titrated upwards to meet the recommended lipid targets. The safety of statin therapy has been well documented (Talbert, 2006); however, fibrates, nicotinic acid, anion exchange resins or ezetimbe can also be offered as an alternative to patients who are insensitive to statin therapy (NICE, 2008).

Summary

Cardiac rehabilitation is an evidence-based approach that focuses on managing patients with CHD through lifestyle interventions and cardioprotective medication. Lifestyle interventions in a CR setting include a supervised, or at home, exercise programme, advice on the Mediterranean diet and in some instances counselling on smoking cessation. In addition, CHD patients should be assessed and, where necessary, treated for anxiety and/or depression. The overall evidence for promoting and implementing the various lifestyle interventions and prescribing cardioprotective medication has been well documented in reducing several CHD risk factors along with reducing cardiac mortality and morbidity. However, when delivering lifestyle interventions social, cultural and financial considerations must always be considered in tailoring treatment to the individual needs of each patient.

References

Ades PA, Savage PD, Toth MJ et al. (2009) High-calorie-expenditure exercise: a new approach to cardiac rehabilitation for overweight coronary patients. Circulation **119**: 2671-8.

American College of Sports Medicine (2005) Guidelines for exercise testing and prescription (7e). London, Lippincott Williams and Wilkins.

Antiplatelet Trialists' Collaboration (1994) Collaborative overview of randomized trials of antiplatelet therapy-I: Prevention of death, myocardial infarction, and stroke by prolonged antiplatelet therapy in various categories of people. Antiplatelet trialists' collaboration. British Medical Journal **308**: 81-106.

Antithrombotic Trialists' Collaboration (2002) Collaborative meta-analysis of randomized trials of antiplatelet therapy for the prevention of death, myocardial infarction, and stroke in high risk people. British Medical Journal **324**: 71-86.

Appel LJ, Moore TJ and Obarzanek E (1997) A clinical trial of the effects of dietary patterns on blood pressure. New England Medical Journal **336**: 1117-24.

Aveyard P and West R (2007) Managing smoking cessation. British Medical Journal **335**: 37-41.

British Association for Cardiac Rehabilitation (BACR) (2007) Standards and Core Components for Cardiac Rehabilitation. Available at www.bcs.com/documents/affiliates/bacr/BACR%20Standards%202007.pdf (accessed July 2008).

British Association for Cardiac Rehabilitation (BACR) (2006) BACR Phase IV Training Module Manual (4e). Leeds, Human Kinetics.

British Association for Cardiac Rehabilitation (BACR) (1995) Guidelines for Cardiac Rehabilitation. London, Blackwell Science.

Baigent C, Keech A, Kearney PM et al. (2005) Efficacy and safety of cholesterol-lowering treatment: prospective meta-analysis of data from 90,056 participants in 14 randomised trials of statins. Lancet **366**: 1267-78.

Beck AT, Ward CH, Mendelson M et al. (1961) An inventory for measuring depression. Archives of General Psychiatry **4**: 53-6.

Borg G (1998) Borg's Perceived Exertion and Pain Scales. Leeds. Human Kinetics.

Brodie D (2000) Cardiac Rehabilitation: An Educational `Resource. London, BACR.

Cannon CP, Braunwald E, McCabe CH et al. for the Pravastatin or Atorvastatin Evaluation and Infection Therapy-Thrombolysis in Myocardial Infarction 22 investigators (2004) Intensive versus moderate lipid lowering with statins after acute coronary syndrome (PROVE-IT). New England Medical Journal **350**: 494-504.

Carney RM, Freedland KE, Rich MW et al. (1993) Ventricular tachycardia and psychiatric depression in patients with coronary artery disease. American Journal of Medicine **95**(1): 23-8.

Carney RM, Rich MW, Tevelde A et al. (1987) Major depressive disorder in coronary heart disease. American Journal of Cardiology **60**: 1273-5.

Clarke AM, Harting L, Vandermeer B et al. (2005) Meta-analysis: secondary prevention programmes for patients with coronary artery disease. Annals of Internal Medicine **143**(9): 659-72.

Davies SJC, Jackson PR, Potokar J et al. (2004) Treatment of anxiety and depressive disorders in patients with cardiovascular disease. Clinical review. British Medical Journal **328**: 939-43.

de Lemos JA, Blazing MA, Wiviott SD et al. (2004) Early intensive vs a delayed conservative simvastatin strategy in people with acute coronary syndromes: phase Z of the A to Z trial. Journal of the American Medical Association **292**: 1307-16.

Department of Health (2004) At Least Five a Week: Evidence on the Impact of Physical Activity and its Relationship to Health. London, Department of Health. Available at www.dh.gov.uk/assetroot/04/08/09/81/04080981.pdf (accessed 20 July 2008).

Department of Health (2000) National Service Frameworks for Coronary Heart Disease. London, Department of Health.

Dickstein K, Cohen-Solal A, Filippatos G et al. (2008) ESC Guidelines for the Diagnosis and Treatment of Acute and Chronic Heart Failure 2008. The Task Force for the Diagnosis and Treatment of Acute and Chronic Heart Failure 2008 of the European Society of Cardiology. Developed in collaboration with the Heart Failure Association of the ESC (HFA) and endorsed by the European Society of Intensive Care Medicine (ESICM). European Heart Journal **29**: 2388-442.

Estruch R, Martínez-González MA, Corella D et al. (2006) Effects of a Mediterranean-style diet on cardiovascular risk factors. a randomized trial. Annals of Internal Medicine **145**: 1-11.

Frasure-Smith N, Lesperance F, Gravel G et al. (2000) Depression and health care costs during the first year following myocardial infarction. Journal of Psychosomatic Research **48**: 471-8.

Freemantle N, Cleland J, Young P et al. (1999) B Blockade after myocardial infarction: systematic review and meta regression analysis. British Medical Journal **318**: 1730-7.

Glassman AH, Bigger T, Gaffney M et al. (2006) Onset of major depression associated with acute coronary syndromes relationship of onset, major depressive disorder history, and episode severity to sertraline benefit. Archives of General Psychiatry **63**: 283-8.

Hambrecht R, Niebauer J, Marburger C et al. (1994) Various intensities of leisure time physical activity in patients with coronary athersclerotic lesions. Journal of the American College of Cardiology **14**: 167-68.

Hippisley-Cox J and Coupland C (2005) Effect of combinations of drugs on all cause mortality in patients with ischaemic heart disease: nested case-control analysis. British Medical Journal **330**: 1059-63.

Kostis JB, Jackson G, Rosen R et al. (2005) Sexual dysfunction and cardiac risk (the Second Princeton Consensus Conference). American Journal of Cardiology **26**: 85M-93M.

Kronish IM, Rieckmann N and Halm EA (2006) Persistent depression affects adherence to secondary prevention behaviors after acute coronary syndromes. Journal of General Internal Medicine **21**(11): 1178-83.

Levitan EB, Wolk A and Mittleman MA (2009) Fish consumption, marine omega-3 fatty acids, and incidence of heart failure: a population-based prospective study of middle-aged and elderly men. European Heart Journal **30**(12): 1495-500.

Lichtman JH, Bigger T Jr and Blumenthal JA (2008) Depression and coronary heart disease. Recommendations for screening, referral, and treatment: a science advisory from the American Heart Association Prevention Committee of the Council on Cardiovascular Nursing, Council on Clinical Cardiology, Council on Epidemiology and Prevention, and Interdisciplinary Council on Quality of Care and Outcomes Research: endorsed by the American Psychiatric Association. *Circulation* **118**: 1768-75.

Linden W, Phillips MJ and Leclerc J (2007) Psychological treatment of cardiac patients: a meta-analysis. *European Heart Journal* **28**: 2972-84.

Logue J, Thompson L, Romanes F, Wilson DC, Thompson J and Sattar N (2010) Management of obesity: summary of SIGN guideline. *British Medical Journal* **340**: 154.

Martínez-González MA, Fernández-Jarne E, Serrano-Martínez M, Wright M and Gomez-Gracia E (2004) Development of a short dietary intake questionnaire for the quantitative estimation of adherence to a cardioprotective Mediterranean diet. *European Journal of Clinical Nutrition* **58**: 1550-2. doi:10.1038/sj. ejcn.1602004.

Mead A, Atkinson D, Albin D *et al.* (2006) Dietetic guidelines on food and nutrition in the secondary prevention of cardiovascular disease evidence from systematic reviews of randomised controlled trials (second update, January 2006). *Journal of Human Nutrition and Diet* **19**: 401-19.

Mensink RP, Zock PL and Kester DM (2003) Effects of dietary fatty acids and carbohydrates on the ratio of serum total to HDL cholesterol and on serum lipids and apolipoproteins: a meta-analysis 60 controlled trials. *American Journal of Clinical Nutrition* **77**: 1146-55.

Milani RV, Lavie CJ and Cassidy MM (1996) Effects of cardiac rehabilitation and exercise training programs on depression in patients after major cardiac events. *American Heart Journal* **132**: 726-32.

Milani RV and Lavie CJ (2007) Impact of cardiac rehabilitation on depression and its associated mortality. *American Journal of Medicine* **120**: 799-806.

National Audit of Cardiac Rehabilitation (NACR) (2008) *Annual Statistical Report 2008.* British Heart Foundation, London. Available at www.cardiacrehabilitation.org.uk/dataset.htm (accessed June 2009).

National Institute for Health and Clinical Excellence (2008) *Lipid Modification: Cardiovascular Risk Assessment and the Modification of Blood Lipids for the Primary and Secondary Prevention of Cardiovascular Disease. Quick Reference Guide*. NICE clinical guideline 67. Available at www.nice.org.uk/nicemedia/pdf/ CG67NICEGuidance.pdf (accessed September 2008).

National Institute for Health and Clinical Excellence (NICE) (2007a) MI: secondary prevention in primary and secondary care for patients following a myocardial infarction. NICE Clinical Guideline 48. Available at www.nice.org.uk/nicemedia/ pdf/CG48NICEGuidance.pdf (accessed July 2008).

National Institute for Health and Clinical Excellence (NICE) (2007b) *Depression (Amended). Management of Depression in Primary and Secondary Care.* NICE Clinical Guideline 23. Available at www.nice.org.uk/nicemedia/pdf/ CG23NICEguidelineamended.pdf (accessed June 2009).

Pollock ML, Lowenthal DT and Foster C (1991) Acute and chronic responses to exercise in patients treated with beta-blockers. *Journal of Cardiopulmonary Rehabilitation* **11**: 132-44.

Quist-Paulsen P and Gallefoss F (2003) Randomised controlled trial of smoking cessation intervention after admission for coronary heart disease. *British Medical Journal* **327**: 1254-8.

Sacks FM, Svetkey LP, Vollmer WM *et al.* (2001) Effects on blood pressure of reduced dietary sodium and the Dietary Approaches to Stop Hypertension (DASH) diet. *New England Medical Journal* **344**: 3-10.

Scandinavian Simvastatin Survival Study Group (1994) Randomised trial of cholesterol lowering in 4444 patients with coronary heart disease: Scandinavian Survival Study (4S). *Lancet* **344**: 1383-9.

Schleifer SJ, Marcari-Hinson MM, Coyle DA *et al.* (1989) The nature and course of depression following myocardial infarction. *Archives of Internal Medicine* **149**: 1785-9.

Schwartz GG, Olsson AG, Ezekowitz MD *et al.* (2001) Effects of atorvastatin on early recurrent ischaemic events in acute coronary syndromes. The MIRACL study: a randomised contolled trial. *Journal of the American Medical Association* **285**: 1711-18.

Scottish Intercollegiate Guidelines Network (SIGN) (2000) *Cardiac Rehabilitation, no. 57.* Edinburgh, SIGN.

Stansfeld SA and Marmot MG (2002) *Stress and the Heart: Psychosocial Pathways to Coronary Heart Disease.* London, BMJ Books.

Talbert RL (2006) Safety issues with statin therapy. *Journal of the American Pharmacists Association.* **46**(4): 479-90.

Trichopoulou A, Christina B and Trichopoulos D (2005) Mediterranean diet and survival among patients with coronary heart disease in Greece. *Archives of Internal Medicine* **165**: 929-35.

Truswell S (2003) *ABC of Nutrition: Reducing the Risk of Coronary Heart Disease.* London, BMJ Books.

van Melle JP, de Jonge P, Spijkerman TA *et al.* (2004) Prognostic association of depression following myocardial infarction with mortality and cardiovascular events: a meta-analysis. *Psychosomatic Medicine* **66**: 814-22.

Vieweg BW and Hedlund JL (1983) The general health questionnaire (GHQ); a comprehensive review. *Journal of Operational Psychiatry* **14**: 74-81.

Williams MA (2004) Exercise testing in cardiac rehabilitation: exercise prescription and beyond. *Cardiology Clinics* **19**: 415-31.

Wood D, Wray R, Poulter N *et al.* (2005) JBS 2: Joint British Societies' guidelines on prevention of cardiovascular disease in clinical practice. *Heart* **91**(supp 5): 1-52.

Yusuf S, Sleight P, Pogue J *et al.* (2000) Effects of an angiotensin-converting-enzyme inhibitor, ramipril, on cardiovascular events in high-risk patients. *The Heart Outcomes Prevention* **342**(18): 1376.

Zigmond AS and Snaith RP (1983) The hospital anxiety and depression scale. *Acta Psychiatrica Scandinavica* **67**: 361-70.

Chapter 15

Ethical Issues in Cardiac Care

Pauline Walsh and Fiona Foxall

Introduction

All nurses working in the cardiac care setting will encounter ethical dilemmas during the course of their work which can evoke anxiety and challenge thinking. Concerns relating to "Do Not Attempt Resuscitation" (DNAR) orders and withdrawal of active treatment can seem difficult to interpret. Sudden, unexpected death is common in cardiac care, but various legal and ethical issues may arise prior to the event. Issues of consent, autonomy and competence are major concerns that are frequently encountered. Nurses, both as distinct practitioners and as part of the multidisciplinary team, make a key contribution to the ethical decision-making process. The aim of this chapter is to increase awareness and understanding of the legal and ethical concerns underpinning the care for patients within cardiac settings.

Learning outcomes

At the end of this chapter the reader will be able to:

- examine ethical decision-making frameworks for use in practice
- discuss the concept of establishing competence
- outline the principles of informed consent
- discuss the ethical concerns surrounding DNAR
- discuss the ethics of withdrawal of active treatment.

Ethical theory and principles in perspective

Ethics is concerned with considering "what one ought to do", in other words what is right or wrong. It is a branch of philosophy often referred to as moral

Nursing the Cardiac Patient, First Edition. Edited by Melanie Humphreys.
© 2011 Blackwell Publishing Ltd. Published 2011 by Blackwell Publishing Ltd.

philosophy and is not unique to healthcare settings. Indeed, ethical deliberation can be traced back to Plato and Aristotle with their teachings of virtue ethics (Park *et al.*, 2003). Changes in medicine and healthcare over the past century have been incredible both in speed and complexity, bringing with them increasing need to make sometimes difficult decisions about what ought to be done. Thus clinicians need an understanding of ethics and skills of ethical reasoning to guide their decision making and help them support their patients and clients in making informed choices. There are many theoretical approaches used within philosophy; however, this chapter will focus on those most commonly associated with healthcare ethics.

There are two major ethical theories that guide healthcare practice. Deontology (duty-based theory), the basic tenet of which is, "I must always carry out my duty"; and utilitarianism (consequence-based theory), which asserts that an action is right if it produces the greatest benefit for the greatest number of people. In reality it is unlikely that anyone would make all decisions based on only one of these theories, they would probably draw on aspects of both. Difficulties in applying the theories to practical issues occur when trying to decide what our duty is or what the greatest benefit is. During the 1960s and 1970s, practitioners found that these broad theories did not provide enough guidance for them when trying to establish the appropriate course of action to take and the field of bioethics emerged. From this came the birth of the principles approach. Within this approach there are four guiding ethical principles.

- **Non-maleficence** – first and above all – do no harm.
- **Beneficence** – do good, promote good, remove evil or harm.
- **Respect for autonomy** – taking into account and acting on the patient's wishes.
- **Justice** – fairness, entitlement or right.

Beauchamp and Childress (2001)

Such principles are established within codes of practice that guide healthcare practitioners (Nursing and Midwifery Council, 2008), although there will be times when it is not immediately clear which principle takes priority. However, these theories and principles can aid decision making by asking six simple questions.

- What is my duty in this particular circumstance?
- By carrying out my duty, will my actions produce the best available consequences for all concerned?
- Will my actions harm anyone, particularly the patient?
- Am I going to do or promote good for those concerned?
- Am I respecting the patient's wishes?
- Are my actions fair to all concerned?

Coming to the right decision will not rest just on the ethical perspective but will also require contextual consideration, e.g. what are the legal and professional frameworks in operation?, as recent cases involving assisted suicide within European countries highlight differences in legal status. Codes of practice for health professionals draw on such ethical theories and principles and provide guidance regarding professional behaviour. The Code of Professional Conduct for Nurses, Midwives and Health Visitors was revised in 2008 and places greater emphasis on respecting autonomy and beneficence (NMC, 2008). Some writers identify a theory-practice gap between the use of normative ethical theories and the reality of practical decision making and argue that other factors relating to local policy and the specifics of a situation should be given consideration (Cooper *et al.*, 2008; Seedhouse 1998). Kirklin (2007) suggests that moral reasoning includes both logic and intuition, and goes on to identify that healthcare professionals may indeed see the effectiveness of an ethical argument, but their intuition causes them to disagree with the suggested outcome, resulting in potential conflict. A number of frameworks to guide ethical reasoning and ultimate decision making have subsequently been developed.

Ethical decision-making frameworks

Best interest model

This model relies heavily on the principle of beneficence as identified above. Central to its premise is that health professionals should act "in a way that most optimally promotes the good of the individual" (Bailey, 2006). The NMC stipulate that nurses "must be able to demonstrate that they acted in the best interest of a client when providing emergency care" (NMC, 2008). It is often associated with situations where the patient does not have capacity to consent, or in an emergency situation where decisions need to be made rapidly with very little available information regarding the context of the patient. Thus the patient admitted to the emergency department in a state of cardiac arrest will be resuscitated on the basis that it is in their best interest to try to preserve life. The Mental Capacity Act (Department for Constitutional Affairs, 2005) provides the legal framework to promote the best interest of those who lack the capacity to make their own decisions.

Four quadrants approach

This approach initially described by Jonsen, categorises the four broad topics of medical intervention, patient preference, quality of life and contextual features, which should be considered when undertaking an ethics case analysis (Jonsen *et al.*, 2006).

Sokol (2008) asserts that the four quadrants approach is an appropriate methodological model for ethical decision making and it would seem to be useful in cardiac situations; however, the potential for the patient to not be fully involved in the decision-making process is always a risk.

The ethical grid

This was developed by David Seedhouse as a tool that applies a holistic approach to the decision-making process. He asks that practitioners when faced with the need to make a decision should identify what they intuitively feel is the correct decision and then use the grid to try to disprove it. The tool requires the decision making to explore each of the layers in the ethical grid in turn (Figure 15.1). While the grid can be looked at either in terms of a flat structure or as a pyramid with the blue layer being at the top, he emphasises that no one layer is more important in its own right than any other and that what is important is the specific situation being considered. Thus when analysing the answers to the questions within each layer the clinician would need to establish their priority in that specific situation and balance them

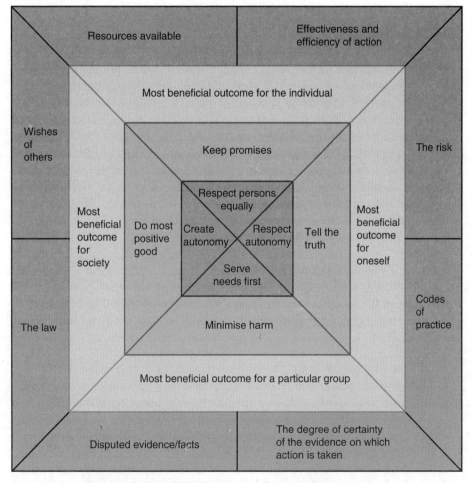

Figure 15.1 The ethical grid. From Seedhouse (1998). Reproduced with permission from John Wiley & Sons.

against each other. The rigour of analysis should then ensure that the most appropriate action is taken.

It is evident that there is a range of decision-making approaches that can help to guide the practitioner in making decisions about nursing care or contributing to the wider decision-making process. While there are differences within each model, what is important is that practitioners undertake reasoned thought processes to ensure that they can justify their actions and to promote the best interests of the patient. Extended technologies and developments in cardiac nursing result in nurses having to increasingly explore ethical issues. The need for contextual analysis is crucial as legal, professional or local service delivery requirements may supersede an ethical view and in fact determine the approach a clinician may take. Indeed, cardiac nurses need to examine their own knowledge and reflect on the situations they face within clinical practice in order to explore the process itself in conjunction with the specific analysis of an individual case.

Informed consent

Patients have fundamental legal and ethical rights in determining what happens to their own bodies (DH, 2001). Consent is simply the agreement of the patient to undergo a proposed form of treatment, although consent which is not based on understanding is not valid consent. For consent to be valid, it needs to be informed, i.e. the patient must understand the proposed treatment. To understand it, the patient must receive an explanation of the procedure and this explanation must be given in a form that is comprehensible to the patient. If alternative forms of treatment are available, these should be discussed; substantial risks and possible consequences of the procedure should also be explained (Dimond, 2005).

Informed consent, therefore, can be described as:

- a voluntary, uncoerced decision
- made by a sufficiently competent or autonomous person
- on the basis of adequate information and deliberation to accept rather than reject some proposed course of action that will affect them (Gillon, 1985).

Consent may be expressed either verbally or in writing, or implied through compliant actions, for example a patient rolling up a sleeve when a practitioner approaches to take a sample of blood. Obtaining written consent is normal practice for invasive and surgical procedures; verbal or implied consent is generally acceptable for non-invasive and non-surgical procedures (Dimond, 2005).

No one may give consent on behalf of an adult unless they have lasting power of attorney (Mental Capacity Act, 2005). If the patient is incompetent, the clinician/health professional (as all are bound by the MCA to act in best interests) can act in the best interests of the patient, or out of necessity, and therefore ignore refusal of consent by a relative. Any proposed treatment is lawful if it is in the best interests of the patient and unlawful if it is not.

DNAR

Cardiopulmonary resuscitation (CPR) is a procedure that attempts to restore cardiac and/or respiratory function to individuals who have sustained a cardiac and/or respiratory arrest. "Do Not Attempt Resuscitation" (DNAR) is a medical order to provide no resuscitation to individuals for whom resuscitation is futile and therefore inappropriate (or who have refused life-saving treatment).

Cardiopulmonary resuscitation has the ability to reverse premature death. It can also prolong terminal illness, increase discomfort and consume enormous resources (Ewanchuck and Brindley, 2006). Only 10–20% of all those in whom CPR is attempted in acute general hospitals will live to be discharged (Bowker and Stewart, 1999). It is therefore clear that CPR is often futile and where possible medical staff will consider a DNAR order.

The important concept here is that of medical futility and refers to interventions that are unlikely to produce any significant benefit for the patient. This can be in terms of either the likelihood that an intervention will benefit the patient or the quality of any benefit that does occur. A treatment that merely produces a physiological effect on a patient's body does not necessarily confer any benefit that the patient can appreciate. The question is "Does the intervention have any reasonable prospect of helping the patient?" (Jecker, 2000).

Wherever possible the decision to not attempt resuscitation should be made by all those involved in the patient's care, the patient's significant others and, most importantly, where the patient is competent to make decisions, the patient themself. In 2007, a joint document from the British Medical Association (BMA), Royal College of Nursing (RCN) and Resuscitation Council of the United Kingdom (RCUK) was published to provide guidance relating to CPR outlining legal and ethical issues to be considered. Key principles within this are the need for CPR decisions to be based on an individual assessment and where possible advanced care planning, which involves good communication and information giving.

In some circumstances patients may have expressed a wish to not be resuscitated or to not have certain types of treatment, known as an advance directive (also referred to as living wills, advance statements or advance refusals). These are usually written directives from competent individuals to healthcare professionals regarding treatment that should be provided or foregone in specific circumstances, during periods of incompetence (Beauchamp and Childress, 2001). However, an advance directive does not have to be written to be valid. If a patient makes a verbal advance statement that they do not wish to have a particular form of treatment, should they become incapacitated, this must be respected. Advance directives are rooted in respect for autonomy, which is one of the foremost ethical principles (Beauchamp and Childress, 2001). Western society places great importance on a person's right to self-determination even when they are unable to participate in decision making due to incompetence (De Wolf Bosek and Savage, 2007). As competent adult patients have a right to refuse medical treatment, an advance directive is a way of prolonging autonomy. However, an advance directive cannot request treatment that is not in the best interests of the patient.

The legality of an advance directive is now covered within the Mental Capacity Act 2005 which came into force in 2007. This act places a responsibility on professionals to uphold the wishes of the patient within the specific circumstances outlined, and is supported by both the BMA and the Nursing and Midwifery Council (NMC).

Where there is any doubt, healthcare professionals should always err on the side of saving life. Practitioners should take into account relatives' wishes during any decision-making process, but in deciding whether or not to resuscitate a patient, these views should not be the only consideration (Dimond, 2005).

The ethics of withdrawal of active treatment

Cardiac care may involve withdrawal of treatment and end-of-life decisions. Difficulties may arise when caring for patients at the end of their lives who are unable to make decisions about continuation of treatment. Ethical dilemmas arise when there is a perceived conflicting duty to the patient, such as a conflict between the duty to preserve life and a duty to act in the patient's best interests, or when an ethical principle such as respect for autonomy conflicts with a duty not to harm. Nurses should use the guidance laid out in the end-of-life care programme to ensure that they provide the best care for patients at the end of their life (DH, 2006). Importantly, practitioners have no obligation to offer treatments or procedures that do not benefit patients. Futile treatments are ill advised because they often increase a patient's pain and discomfort in the last days and weeks of life, and because they can expend finite medical resources (Jecker, 2000).

The principle of beneficence is a moral obligation to act to benefit others or to act in the best interests of others. In healthcare, this may seem obvious as an obligation, but there is a risk that we can begin to believe we know what is best for them. In our wish to do good for the patient, we can override their autonomy and step beyond the boundary of beneficence into paternalism, i.e. the overriding of one person's preferences by another person and possibly inflict harm.

The ethical principle of non-maleficence, the obligation not to inflict harm intentionally, is important here. Many treatments and procedures in healthcare cause harmful side effects, but the interventions save or improve quality of life overall. However, there are times when a patient's quality of life is so poor or the intervention would prove so burdensome that it is more appropriate to withhold or withdraw it, as the balance of harm over benefit is too great. The major considerations in end-of-life decision making is the degree of harm being caused by the interventions, whether that harm outweighs any benefits and, indeed, whether death would be a harm in the circumstances.

It is justifiable to discontinue life-sustaining treatments if:

- the patient has the ability to make decisions, fully understands the consequences of their decision and states they no longer want a treatment
- the treatment no longer offers benefit to the patient (Braddock, 1999).

Although many practitioners feel it is more acceptable to not start a treatment rather than to withdraw it, there is actually no ethical distinction between withholding and withdrawing treatment (Beauchamp and Childress, 2001; Braddock, 1999).

Patients' rights and responsibilities

The NHS was established in 1948 to afford people the right to receive healthcare free at the point of delivery. Since then the concept of patients' rights has continued to develop to not only include having access to free care, but also to having a say in the way that care is actually provided. Respect for and promotion of patient autonomy is now a central component of Department of Health guidance relating to consent to treatment and professional body codes of practice. Thompson *et al.* (2006) identify different types of rights that outline what is to occur or to whom it occurs:

- *positive* – implies a right to an action
- *negative* – implies a lack of action
- *particular* – to an individual
- *universal* – can be seen as a general rule.

In addition to this, Leathard and McLaren (2007) discuss that rights can be considered as concrete/fundamental; those that are based in law, for example international human rights; and those that are aspirational – what we would strive for. With ever-increasing advances in medicine, technologies and therapeutic interventions, questions are being raised relating to patients' rights to specific types of treatment and care. The NHS has devolved the commissioning of patient services to primary care trusts (PCTs) which must consider the best way of allocating its resources. High-profile cases relating to the refusal of PCTs to permit the use of drugs for the treatment of cancer or degenerative neurological disorders have fuelled the debate both within the professional and political arena.

Box 15.1   Patients' rights versus responsibilities –
a case study

James is a 50-year-old man with cardiovascular disease who has a
wife and four children, two of whom are still at school. He has been
experiencing significant symptoms, including pain, breathlessness and
fatigue from his disease, and is now unable to continue with his job
as a builder. He takes very little physical activity and has become
socially isolated resulting in periods of depression.

The cardiac nurse visits James at home on a regular basis and is
trying to encourage him to make important lifestyle changes as he
smokes 30 cigarettes a day and has a very poor diet that is high in
fatty foods.

James does not want to make these changes and feels that he
should be given all the possible treatments available without people
trying to interfere in how he chooses to live his life.

Should there be responsibilities associated with rights?

Patients' rights versus responsibilities – review the following case study
(Box 15.1).

Discussion

It is clear that the nurse has a duty of care to James and that he has a right
to healthcare services; however, what this means is less clear. Approaches
can be considered from different standpoints as punitive or non- punitive.
If a punitive stance is taken then James's refusal to change his lifestyle
could be seen as a refusal to take responsibility for his actions and may
reduce his claim on rights to healthcare. Indeed many surgeons require
patients to reduce weight or the number of cigarettes smoked to a certain
point before they will agree to go ahead with surgery. This may be considered a sensible clinical approach in order to reduce the risk of complications,
or a punishment for causing their own ill health. A non-punitive stance
may assert that James has a legitimate claim on rights to healthcare and as
such should be provided with the treatment regardless of whether he stops
smoking.

The NMC code of conduct (2008) infers a duty on nurses to provide care
in a non-discriminatory way, which implies that they should direct interventions to empower patients to make appropriate healthy life choices. Thus in
this situation, the nurse has a challenging situation to continue to try to
provide health promotion and support to James, while respecting his
autonomy.

Summary

As nurses expand their scope of practice and technology continues to advance, it is inevitable that all nurses working in the cardiac care setting will encounter ethical dilemmas during the course of their practice. This chapter has examined some of the key models for ethical practice that will serve as a useful framework for the cardiac nurse. Issues regarding consent, DNAR and withdrawing treatment have also being explored. Cardiac care nurses need to embrace insightful ethical practice both as distinct practitioners and as part of the multidisciplinary team, as they will continue to make a key contribution to the ethical decision-making process relating to the care of their patients.

References

Bailey S (2006) Decision making in acute care: a practical framework supporting the bests interests principle. *Nursing Ethics* **13**(3): 284-91.

Beauchamp TL and Childress JF (2001) *Principles of Biomedical Ethics (5e)*. Oxford, Oxford University Press.

Bowker L and Stewart K (1999) Predicting unsuccessful cardiopulmonary resuscitation (CPR): a comparison of three morbidity scores. *Resuscitation* **40**: 89-95.

Braddock CH (1999) *Termination of Life-Sustaining Treatment* http://dets.washington.edu/bioethx/topics/termlife.html (accessed 27 April 2007).

Cooper R, Bissell P and Wingfield J (2008) Ethical decision-making, passivity and pharmacy. *Journal of Medical Ethics* **34**: 441-5.

Department for Constitutional Affairs (2005) *Mental Capacity Act: Code of Practice*. London, The Stationery Office.

Department of Health (2006) *NHS End of Life Care Programme Progress Report*. London, HMSO.

Department of Health (2001) *Reference Guide to Consent for Examination or Treatment*. London, HMSO.

De Wolf Bosek MS and Savage TA (2007) *The Ethical Component of Nursing Education: Integrating Ethics into Clinical Experience*. London, Lippincott.

Dimond B (2005) *Legal Aspects of Nursing (4e)*. Harlow, Pearson Longman.

Ewanchuck M and Brindley PG (2006) Ethics review: Perioperative do-not-resuscitate orders – doing "nothing" when something can be done. www.ccforum.com (accessed 15 April 2007).

Gillon R (1985) *Philosophical Medical Ethics*. Chichester, Wiley.

Jecker NS (2000) Futility. http://depts.washington.edu/bioethx/topics/futil.html (accessed 27 April 2007).

Jonsen A, Siegler M and Windslade W (2006) *Clinical Ethics (6e)*. New York, McGraw-Hill.

Kirklin D (2007) Minding the gap between logic and intuition: an interpretative approach to ethical analysis. *Journal of Medical Ethics* **33**: 386-9.

Leathard A and McLaren S (eds) (2007) *Ethics: Contemporary Challenges in Health and Social Care*. Bristol, Policy Press.

Nursing and Midwifery Council (2008) *The Code: Standards of Conduct Performance and Ethics for Nurses*. London, NMC.

Park H, Cameron M, Han S, Ahn S, Oh H and Kim K (2003) Korean nursing students' ethical problems and ethical decision making. *Nursing Ethics* **10**(6): 638-53.

Seedhouse D (1998) *Ethics: The Heart of Healthcare (2e)*. London, John Wiley and Sons.

Sokol D (2008) The "Four Quadrants" approach to clinical ethics case analysis; an application and review. *Journal of Medical Ethics* **34**: 513-16.

Thompson I, Melia M, Botd K and Horsburg D (2006) *Nursing Ethics (5e)*. London, Churchill Livingstone.

Web resources

www.dca.gov.uk/menincap/legis.htm
www.opsi.gov.uk/acts/acts2005/20050009.htm

Appendix A
Patient Transfer to Theatre/ Specialist Centre

Sarah Dickie

Introduction

The decision to transport a critically ill patient, either within a hospital site or to another facility, is based on an assessment of the potential benefits of the transfer weighed against any potential risks. It is a clinical judgement based on physiological variables, concurrent treatment and clinical assessment (NICE, 2007). The decision to transfer a patient must be made by a consultant from the relevant specialties in both the referring and receiving hospitals. Risks to patients may arise from the potential deterioration of the underlying medical condition, the physiological effects of movement, and changes in barometric pressure and temperature associated with air transport (Intensive Care Society, 2002). Benefits will be clear where life-saving interventions are to be performed at the receiving hospital.

Learning outcomes

At the end of this section the reader will be able to:

- describe the steps involved in the preparation of a patient for transfer
- outline the factors to consider when selecting the mode of transport.

Transfer in perspective

Patients are usually transferred to alternative locations for a variety of reasons; these predominantly centre around the need to obtain additional

Nursing the Cardiac Patient, First Edition. Edited by Melanie Humphreys.
© 2011 Blackwell Publishing Ltd. Published 2011 by Blackwell Publishing Ltd.

care that is not currently available at the existing location (Gray *et al.*, 2003), and include:

- no critical care facility on site
- no staffed critical care bed available currently at referring site
- require medical expertise currently unavailable on site
- require specialist facilities
- require investigational facilities
- repatriation.

The transfer of a cardiac patient may be technical, cognitive or procedural in nature, and may involve the patient being transferred to a diagnostic department, operating room or specialised care unit in the hospital. Alternatively, the patient may need to be transferred to a tertiary unit at another hospital to receive this additional care. Around 5,000 cardiac patients require transfer each month in England (Heart Improvement Programme, 2007). The range of transfers include but are not limited to: interhospital transfers of patients with acute coronary syndromes for angiography and revascularisation; transfer from a district general hospital for percutaneous coronary intervention (PCI) or coronary artery bypass surgery; and other emergency or urgent cardiac surgery, for example aortic dissection, urgent valve surgery and implantable cardiac devices.

Critically ill patients are at increased risk of morbidity and mortality during transport (Intensive Care Society, 2002). Risks associated with the timing of transfer and in particular those occurring in the out of hours periods have been shown to have an impact of health outcomes (NICE, 2007) These risks can be minimised and outcomes improved with careful planning and preparation using a systematic approach.

The aim of any transfer is to ensure that the right patient is taken at the right time by the right people to the right place by the right form of transport and receives the right care throughout the journey (Advanced Life support Group, 2002). Interhospital transfers are clearly complex and require a high degree of cross-organisational co-operation. The NHS Heart Improvement Programme has published a number of key documents to provide an underpinning framework to share redesign techniques to improve the efficiency of the non-elective transfer process and the experience for staff and patients (*Signposts to Improving Cardiac Interhospital Transfers* 2007; *Making Moves*, 2006; and *Top Tips to Address Delays for Interhospital Transfers in Cardiac Services*, 2005).

Preparation of the patient for intrahospital or interhospital transfer

Meticulous resuscitation and stabilisation of the patient should be carried out prior to any transfer, regardless of whether the patient is being transferred within the hospital or to a tertiary specialist centre. This is to ensure that the patient transfer proceeds with the minimal change in the level of care provided and to avoid patient deterioration on route. Preparation involves the stabilisation of the patient and measures to ensure the security and safety of the patient during transportation, the preparation of the transfer team personnel and preparation of equipment (Intensive Care Society, 2002).

Patient preparation

The standard ABCDE approach (as detailed in Chapter 11) to patient preparation is essential to ensure that the patient is in the best possible condition prior to the transfer-taking place.

Airway

The airway should be assessed and if necessary secured and protected. Intubating a patient in transit is difficult, so if there is any doubt about the patient's airway or conscious level then elective intubation should be undertaken before departure (Wallace and Ridley, 1999).

Breathing

A patient airway does not ensure adequate ventilation. A full chest examination should be performed again to ensure no life-threatening respiratory conditions have developed. In patients who are spontaneously breathing administer oxygen therapy as indicated via the appropriate oxygen delivery device. Adequacy of respiratory support can be assed by using pulse oximetry and/or capnography.

Oxygen supply can be one of the greatest problems during longer transfers. A simple oxygen consumption calculation should be made prior to departure, based on the flow rate or minute volume of the patient and the anticipated journey time plus 30 minutes' reserve (Advanced Life Support Group, 2002).

$$\text{Predicated journey time} \times \text{Minute volume} =$$
$$\text{Estimated oxygen requirements (minutes)}$$

The number of oxygen cylinders required can then be calculated by dividing the estimated oxygen requirements by the cylinder capacity.

Remember that most portable ventilators are oxygen-driven, providing either 100% oxygen or an air mix. Most ventilators will use 1l/min as a "driving gas". This should be factored into your calculations.

Circulation

Secure venous access, at a minimum of two reliable sites, should be available. To maintain satisfactory blood pressure, perfusion and urine output, intravenous volume loading will usually be required. Unstable patients may need pulmonary artery pressure or central venous pressure monitoring established to optimise filling pressures. A patient who remains persistently hypotensive despite resuscitation should not be moved until sources of any blood loss or sepsis have been identified and controlled. Hypovolaemic patients tolerate transfer poorly, and circulating blood volume should be as near to normal as possible (Intensive Care Society, 2002; Wallace and Ridley, 1999).

Disability

Continue to monitor the conscious level as a response to ongoing resuscitation. Conscious patients should be kept informed of the transfer and all other relevant information.

Exposure

Patients frequently become relatively hypothermic while being stabilised for transfer (Advanced Life Support Group, 2002). Patients should be laid on and wrapped in insulating cellular blankets and then covered with further blankets or duvets to prevent further heat loss. Ensure that access to and visibility of intravenous access and main fluid lines are maintained. All equipment should be securely stored by fastening to the transport trolley (Intensive Care Society, 2002). Under no circumstances should equipment be placed on top of the patient. This may become a dangerous projectile in the event of sudden deceleration.

Clear records must be maintained at all times throughout the transfer and on arrival at the receiving unit. There needs to be clear evidence of continuity of care delivered through a formal structured handover (see Box A.1), supported by a written plan. A written record of the patient status, monitored values, treatment given and any other clinically relevant information should be completed during the transfer (NICE, 2007).

The Scottish Patient Safety Alliance (2008) also recommends the SBAR tool. This was devised to help healthcare providers communicate effectively about a patient's condition.

Box A.1 Recommendations for formal structured handover

- A summary of care, including diagnosis and treatment
- A monitoring and investigation plan
- A plan for ongoing treatment, including drugs and therapies, infection status and any agreed limitations of treatment
- Physical, psychological and emotional needs
- Specific communication or language needs

S - situation

B - background

A - assessment

R - recommendation.

Different members of the team have different communication styles, and have been trained to pass on information in different ways. To improve communication and avoid adverse outcomes for patients, SBAR can be used as a framework to help with getting the right information across.

Equipment preparation

Ideal circumstances would allow the provision of dedicated transfer equipment, which would be stored in a specific location ready charged and regularly checked. A basic equipment list may be helpful to ensure that everything is available and ready for use (Box A.2).

Case notes, X-rays if digital images not available, referral letters, investigation reports and any blood or blood products should be prepared to go with the patient. Before leaving, the travel arrangements should be discussed with relatives and they should be given the opportunity to see the patient. Relatives would not normally travel with the patient in the ambulance. Named medical and nursing personal should also be contacted at the receiving unit to confirm the exact location for the patient, update them on the patient's clinical condition and give them an estimated time of arrival (Advanced Life Support Group, 2002; Intensive Care Society, 2002)

Individual members of the transfer team require personal equipment. A simple checklist mnemonic can be useful as an aide-mémoire (Advanced Life Support Group, 2002) (Box A.3).

Box A.2 Essential patient equipment

- Equipment for basic and advanced airway management, sized appropriately for the patient
- Yankauer sucker and assorted sizes of suction catheter
- Adequate sedation and inotropes
- Oxygen source ample supply for the total journey time plus 30 minutes' reserve
- Additional intravenous access
- Blood pressure monitoring
- Pulse oximeter/capnography.
- Cardiac monitor/defibrillator attached and working
- Drugs, pumps, lines rationalised and secured
- Resuscitation drugs such as adrenaline
- Case notes/X-rays

Box A.3   Essential staff equipment

P	Phone
E	Enquiry number and name
R	Revenue
S	Safe clothing
O	Organised route
N	Nutrition
A	A–Z
L	Lift home

All the transport team must be adequately prepared. Direct telephone contacts allows for seamless communication with both the receiving unit and home unit. Ensure you have some money with you in case of an emergency. Protective clothing should be appropriate to the situation. If the transfer is being undertaken by an ambulance crew unfamiliar with the area or the transfer involves taking the patient outwith the region, ensure that travel directions have been confirmed and take an A–Z with you. Your wellbeing as a healthcare provider is also important, so ensure that your hydration is maintained. Finally, do not assume that you will be automatically brought back to your base hospital by the ambulance crew – have an alternative plan for returning.

Personnel preparation

All individuals involved in the transfer of critically ill patients should be suitably trained and experienced. This can be best achieved through competency-based assessments (Intensive Care Society, 2002). Generally speaking the same level of training is required whether transporting patients between departments within a hospital or between hospitals. However, the skills and competencies required on an inward journey or pre-intervention may differ from those required for an outward or post-intervention journey.

It is recommended that a minimum of two people in addition to the ambulance driver or pilot accompany a critically ill patient during transfer (Intensive Care Society, 2002). Consider what function the escort will provide; for example, support for non-ventilated stable patients or advanced medical or nursing skills. The precise requirements for accompanying personnel will depend on the clinical circumstances in each case. Whatever the category of patient, all personnel should be competent in transfer procedures and be familiar with the clinical condition of the patient and the equipment the patient requires during the transfer journey. Provision must be made for adequate insurance to cover the death or disability of attendants in an accident during the course of their duties (Wallace and Ridley, 1999).

> ## Box A.4   Factors affecting mode of transport
>
> - Nature of illness
> - Urgency of transfer
> - Mobilisation time
> - Geographical factors
> - Availability of transport
> - Traffic and weather conditions
> - Cost

Transport mode

Road ambulances are the most common means of patient transport used in the UK. Road transport also has the advantage of rapid mobilisation times, less disruption from adverse weather conditions, easier patient monitoring with less potential for physiological disturbance and low overall costs. In addition, staff are likely to be more familiar with this type of environment. Air transport should be considered for longer journeys (more than 50 miles or two hours), where road access is difficult, or where for other reasons it may simply be quicker. The perceived speed of air transport should be balanced against the inter-vehicle transfers at either end of the journey and any organisational delays.

For all patient transport decision close liaison with the local ambulance service is essential.

The selection of the most appropriate transport mode should take into account the factors in Box A.4.

Summary

Patient outcomes from interhospital transfer depend to a large degree on the expertise of the personnel and the available technology within each healthcare facility. Regular audit of transfers is necessary to maintain and improve standards. Remember that the aim of any transfer is to ensure that the right patient is taken at the right time by the right people to the right place by the right form of transport and receives the right care throughout the journey (Advanced Life Support Group, 2002).

References

Advanced Life Support Group (2002) *Safe Transfer and Retrieval: The Practical Approach*. London, BMJ Books.

Gray A, Gill S, Airey M and Williams R (2003) Descriptive epidemiology of adult critical care transfers from the emergency department. *Emergency Medicine Journal* **20**: 242-6.

Heart Improvement Programme (2007) *Signposts to Improving Cardiac Interhospital Transfers*. Leicester, NHS Heart Improvement Programme, HIP022; www.heart.nhs.uk

Heart Improvement Programme (2006) *Making Moves: Results of a Data Audit and Review of Service Improvements in Interhospital Transfer Arrangements for Cardiac Patients*. Leicester, NHS Heart Improvement Programme. www.heart.nhs.uk

Heart Improvement Programme (2005) *Top Tips to Address Delays for Interhospital Transfers in Cardiac Services*. Leicester, NHS Heart Improvement Programme. www.dscn.nhs.uk/documents/toptipsinterhospital.pdf

Intensive Care Society (2002) *Guidelines for the Transport of the Critically Ill Adult*. London, Intensive Care Society.

National Institute for Health and Clinical Excellence (2007) *Acutely Ill Patients in Hospital*. NICE Clinical Guideline 50.

Scottish Patient Safety Alliance (2008) *Patient Safety Programme*. Scotland, Institute for Healthcare Improvement

Wallace PGM and Ridley SA (1999) ABC of intensive care: transport of critically ill patients. *British Medical Journal* **319**: 368-71.

Appendix B
Cardiac Rehabilitation Circuit Class

Tim Grove

Class management

Level one

- The participant alternates between cardiovascular (CV) stations on the outside of the circuit with active recovery (AR) stations on the inside of the circuit (moving from capital letter to the same small letter (e.g. A-a, B-b, C-c, D-d, E-e).
- The participant performs one minute on the CV stations and performs 10-15 repetitions on the AR stations.
- The circuit is completed twice.

Level two

- The participant alternates every two CV stations with one active recovery station (e.g. ratio 2:1 A-B-b). The ratio may be progressed every one to two sessions until the participant can complete two complete circuits of CV (e.g. A-B-C-c, A-B-C-D-d, A-B-C-D-E).
- Once the participant can complete two circuits of complete CV stations, intensity can be increased in accordance with heart rate training zones and ratings of perceived exertion (RPE) scores.

Staffing ratios

There should be one member of staff to every five patients and a typical class might have 15 patients (BACR, 2006). The staff may be organised to supervise all aspects of the circuit. For instance, one member of staff might

Nursing the Cardiac Patient, First Edition. Edited by Melanie Humphreys.
© 2011 Blackwell Publishing Ltd. Published 2011 by Blackwell Publishing Ltd.

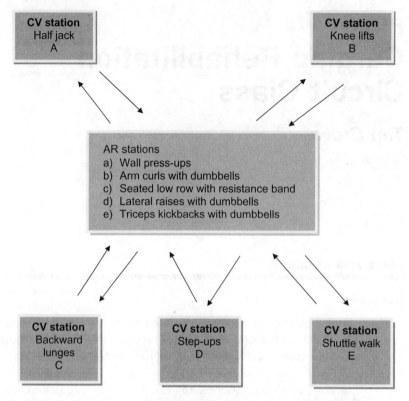

Figure B.1 Cardiac rehabilitation circuit class (adapted with permission from BACR 2006). CV = cardiovascular; AR = active recovery.

be situated in the middle of the AR stations to check exercise technique and to make sure the patient moves on to the correct CV station. One member of staff might circulate around the CV stations to check exercise technique and monitor heart rates and RPE, and the third member of staff might oversee the whole programme and monitor the time spent on each station.

Other considerations

The circuit-based approach permits some participants to adopt an interval approach, while others can undertake continuous aerobic training. It offers a variety of exercise that can be adapted to accommodate individual needs and abilities, as well as allowing individuals to progress at their own rate, both within and between stations (BACR, 2006). The above circuit is simple and uses minimal equipment, which is ideal for cardiac services with limited financial resources, and it can also be used as a template for a home-based exercise programme. However, the circuit can be adapted so that gym equipment (e.g. bikes and rowers) can be used. The bikes and rowers can replace some of the CV stations and might be better-tolerated modes of exercise for patients who are obese or who may suffer from intermittent claudication.

Reference

British Association for Cardiac Rehabilitation (BACR) (2006) *BACR Phase IV Training Module Manual* (4ed). Leeds, Human Kinetics.

Appendix C
Cardiac Pacemakers

Ian Jones and Anne Dormer

Indications and usage

As people live longer their likelihood of suffering from a long-term illness increases. The management of these illnesses takes many forms. The most common medical treatment is the use of drug therapy. However, as technology has increased, alternative means of therapy have been developed. The pacemaker has been used as a means of regulating the heartbeat for many years, but its capability has increased dramatically over recent years with around 25,000 permanent pacemakers being implanted annually in the UK (NICE, 2005). Historically, the pacemaker was used only to pace the ventricles during episodes of complete heart block. However, as computer technology has improved the medical team is now able to implant pacemaker leads into both the atria and ventricles, therefore it can now be used for a wide variety of arrhythmias (Box C.1). These leads, instead of being passive conductors of electrical activity, are now able to sense activity and transmit data back to the pacemaker's own computer. This allows the co-ordination of activity between the atria and ventricles thus improving cardiac output.

Pacemaker function

Pacemakers provide life-saving therapy for some patients and the reduction of symptoms in others. The device works by a generator box producing an electrical impulse, which is relayed down into the chambers of the heart via an electrical lead. The distal end of this lead is implanted into the wall of the chamber of the heart that it is serving. The cardiac cells close to the tip of the lead subsequently transmit this electrical impulse to neighbouring cells and cardiac conduction is initiated.

Nursing the Cardiac Patient, First Edition. Edited by Melanie Humphreys.
© 2011 Blackwell Publishing Ltd. Published 2011 by Blackwell Publishing Ltd.

Box C.1 Indications for insertion of permanent pacemakers

- Heart block: including sinoatrial (SA) block, complete atrioventricular (AV) block, Mobitz type II, trifasicular block
- Symptomatic bradycardia
- Sick sinus syndrome
- Ventricular standstill
- Hypertrophic cardiomyopathy
- Dilated cardiomyopathy
- Long QT syndrome
- Paroxysmal atrial fibrillation (AF) (refractory to drug therapy)
- Tachy-brady syndrome
- Pause-dependent VT
- Ventricular pauses
- Syncope

The pacemakers are also able to sense when the patient's own heart is producing activity and therefore the pacemaker may fall silent and allow the normal conduction to take its course. Alternatively, if a lead in the atria produces a beat in the absence of SA node activity and this impulse travels via the AV node to the ventricles, then the ventricular lead would sense this activity and fall silent, allowing normal AV conduction to occur. Conversely, if the impulse was not transmitted to the ventricles due to AV block, then the lead would produce an electrical stimulus.

The importance of AV synchrony cannot be under estimated. Clearly when conceived, the pacemaker's role was to produce ventricular activity when this was naturally absent. However, due to the improvements in technology, modern-day pacemakers can be programmed to ensure that the atria and ventricles are synchronised. This ultimately improved cardiac output.

NASPE/BPEG code

The pacing mode chosen is described by five letters. These were standardised by the North American Society of Pacing and Electrophysiology (NASPE) and its British equivalent the British Pacing and Electrophysiology group (BPEG). The first letter refers to the chamber of the heart that is being paced. The choice here is obviously either A for atria, V for ventricle or D for dual, where both chambers are being paced. The second letter refers to the chambers of the heart from which the impulse is sensed. Therefore the same letters of A, V or D are used in addition to O, which refers to the absence of the sensing mechanism. This sensing mechanism refers to the situation whereby the lead detects an impulse being produced either naturally from

Table C.1 13 NASPE/BPEG pacemaker codes

Position	I	II	III	IV	V
Category	Chamber paced	Chamber sensed	Response to setting	Programmability	Anti-tachy arrhythmia function
Letter used	O = none A = atrium V = ventricle D = dual	O = none A = atrium V = ventricle D = dual	O = none T = triggered I = inhibited D = dual	O = none P = simple programme M = multiprogramme C = communicating R = rate modulation	O = none P = pacing S = shock D = shock and pacing

the patient's own heart or from the other lead. Once an impulse is sensed the data are transmitted back to the pacemaker's computer and subsequent impulses are controlled. The third letter refers to the pacemaker's response to a sensed impulse. These responses can be either no response (O), triggered (T), inhibited (I), or both triggered and inhibited (T + I). The fourth letter refers to the programmability of the device, which includes features such as rate modulation of the pacemaker. That is, does the pacemaker respond to the patient's need for a faster heart rate such as when exercising. The fifth letter refers to the anti-tachyarrhythmia function. The codes and features are outlined in Table C.1).

Reference

National Institute for Health and Clinical Excellence (2005) *Dual-chamber Pacemakers for Symptomatic Bradycardia due to Sick Sinus Syndrome and/or Atrioventricular Block [Technology appraisal 88]*. London, NICE.

Index

Please note: "ACS" refers to the umbrella term "acute coronary syndromes"

Nursing the Cardiac Patient, First Edition. Edited by Melanie Humphreys.
© 2011 Blackwell Publishing Ltd. Published 2011 by Blackwell Publishing Ltd.